5-Minute
Massage

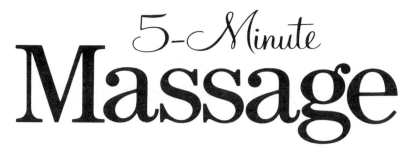

5-Minute Massage

Quick & Simple Exercises to Reduce Tension & Stress

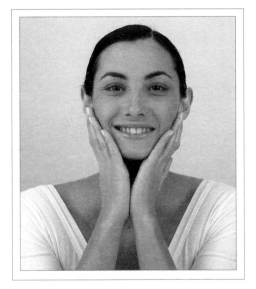

Robert Thé

Sterling Publishing Co., Inc. New York

Photography: Roderick Field
Models: Adéniké Forbes,
Miguel Buss, Janine Dearlove
Make-up by Elisa Johnson

For Virgin Publishing: Carolyn Price

Art direction by Slatter-Anderson
Design by Paul Kime

Library of Congress Cataloging-in-
Publication Data Available

10 9 8 7 6 5 4 3 2

Published 1995 by
Sterling Publishing Company, Inc.
387 Park Avenue South,
New York, N.Y. 10016

Originally published by Virgin Books,
an imprint of Virgin Publishing Ltd
under the title *Stressbusters Five Minute
Massage: Quick and simple techniques for
busy people*

© 1995 by Robert Thé and
Stressbusters/Virgin Publishing Ltd.

Distributed in Canada by
Sterling Publishing
c/o Canadian Nanda Group,
One Atlantic Avenue, Suite 105
Toronto, Ontario, Canada M6K 3E7

Manufactured in the U.S.A.

ISBN: 0-8069-4200-2

This book is dedicated:

To my teachers, clients and students who taught me.
To my friends and colleagues who inspired me.

Special thanks must also go to the following who contributed and participated in the creation of this book: Rosa Amoroso, Alisdair Burcher, Miguel Buss, Malachy Conlan, Diana's Diner, Roderick Field, Adéniké Forbes, Elisa Johnson, Wendy Chalmers-Mill, Christina and Kitsa Pateras, Carolyn Price, Paresh Rink, Dolores Serrallé, Martin Stollery and Joshua Wright.

To you all I give my most heartfelt thanks.

Robert Thé
Covent Garden London
January 1995

*Stressbusters are the UK's leading On-Site Massage company. If you would like
details of corporate services or massage training courses, please contact:
Garden Studios, 11–15 Betterton Street, Covent Garden,
London WC2H 9BP, England. Tel: 0171 379 0344.*

C O N T E N T S

$\mathcal{T}$he Big Picture

Watch any young child at play and you will see a ball of energy, 360° of pure movement, exploding with a combination of grace, power and suppleness as they explore the world around them. Twenty years on and it might be a little difficult to recognize that same child as they stumble out of bed, desperate for a strong coffee, and later return from work to slump in front of the TV, exhausted, suffering from backache, only to nod off in the middle of their favourite programme.

Maybe you can identify with elements in this scenario – you wouldn't be alone. More and more of us are finding that we are increasingly succumbing to the two major problems of living in a fast-moving world; loss of flexibility and stress. Although slow in their effect, they can be thought of as silent epidemics, which go largely unrecognized and unchallenged, yet wreak untold damage in people's lives.

This book aims to change that.

But how is it possible that we go from being children, full of energy and free in our bodies to stiff, aching, tired adults? The answer is progress. As our society has become increasingly sophisticated, we have used our minds more and more and our bodies less and less, so that even the simplest household chore which used to require a high level of physical activity has long since been replaced by a 'labour-saving' device, requiring at most a flick of the wrist. Simply put, at no time in recorded history have we under-used our bodies to this extent.

Whereas most kids 50 years ago would have compensated for being stuck behind a desk all day by playing outdoor games after school, our children today are much more likely to come back home to spend many hours slumped in front of a TV or hunched in front of a computer console. By the time they are ready to join adult society, they will already have begun the process of losing flexibility and bodily awareness, which can rapidly cause a cycle of tension and tiredness.

Yet our bodies are built for movement, and actually require it for optimum performance. Take the shoulder, for example, it has the greatest degree of flexibility of all the joints in the body because several muscles overlap and glide over each other, permitting free and dynamic movement. However, if the shoulder isn't used enough, then these muscles begin to 'stick' to each other, which restricts further movement. This not only affects the immediate area, but also influences the suppleness of the whole body, limiting our movements, and resulting in a gradual loss of flexibility.

But is this whole process inevitable? Do we necessarily have to slow down and lose our agility as we get older? We tend to assume we do because we see so much evidence for it in the form of our own experience and that of people around us. In traditional societies, however, many of the conditions we normally associate with getting older are the exception rather than the norm. In China, for example, many elderly people can be seen at dawn performing martial arts or dancing with a degree of sprightliness and skill that would put many a Western teenager to shame.

The common factor in these societies would seem to be a high degree of physical movement during all stages of life, be it physical work or exercising. It is movement that keeps the body supple and energized, which implies that the ageing process can be greatly affected by the degree to which we use or *fail* to use our bodies throughout our lives. Once this is understood, the choice of whether we lose our physical mobility and energy or whether we remain fluid and dynamic as we get older is one we can consciously make for ourselves.

Life in a fast-moving world also brings with it the problem of stress, which affects each and everyone of us and is becoming increasingly serious. In itself stress is neither good nor bad: it is our reactions to any given situation that are important. What might be a stressful situation for one person, may be quite pleasurable for another. What one person may see as too much work and a headache, another might see as a challenge and opportunity to thrive. We all need different levels of activity and stimulus.

What is important, though, is that we learn to strike the right balance between keeping busy and learning how to relax. Many people get the first part right and lead full, active lives, but they often forget about the second part which is just as important. Unfortunately, our society teaches us that it is good to be busy and somehow sinful and lazy to relax, and we're now reaching a point where more and more people are ending up in hospital with stress-related illnesses simply because they did not know how to or were unable to relax. For example, if you took a Ferrari, one of the world's best sportscars, and drove it non-stop for several years at high speed, without rest or regular servicing, it would eventually develop faults and perhaps even break down completely. Our bodies are no different. Yes, it's good to slip into fifth gear every so often, but it's also important to learn how to switch the ignition off.

You can get a clear idea of what continual, relentless stress and tension feels like by clenching your fist and holding it straight out in front of you. Soon your arm will begin to ache, then quiver and then become painful until you are unable to keep it up any longer. Yet this is the same level of tension that we all carry in our bodies when our muscles are tight, that drains our energy and can age us prematurely.

In the 1980s aerobic exercise was presented as a complete solution to all these problems. Certainly, movement is good for the body but more often than not exercise does little to increase flexibility,

often leaving people with stiffer not suppler muscles. Furthermore, although exercise is a good way of releasing tension, it is not the same as relaxing; far from being a complete solution, it is only a partial answer.

So how can we become more flexible, relaxed and vibrantly alive?

𝒯he Solution

More and more people are asking themselves this question and have begun to search for simple and natural ways to remain in optimum health. Many are finding that massage, which has been used for centuries, is the most effective solution for remaining supple and relaxed in a stressful world. This has created an explosion in its popularity over the past decade as its many benefits are rediscovered.

Unfortunately, the very people who could most benefit from regular massage – people with busy and hectic lifestyles – are those with the least time and opportunity to experience it.

This is why the Five Minute Massage has been developed: to allow busy people the chance to enjoy all the benefits of massage anytime, anywhere – at home, in the office or even while travelling. In order to do so, we have drawn on our extensive experience and from many traditions around the world to create short, simple self-massage sequences which can help to:

- reduce stress and tension
- increase your flexibility and bodily awareness
- calm and relax your nervous system
- improve the circulation of blood
- activate your body's own self-healing mechanisms
- boost your energy levels
- take years off you
- help you to feel vibrantly alive.

Self-massage is our most basic instinct which allows us not only to relax contracted muscles and improve the flow of energy through our bodies, but also to discover things we never knew about ourselves: where we ache, or are stiff, and what sort of techniques and pressures we enjoy.

These massage sequences are simple to learn, involve no undressing, and are highly effective, providing the maximum benefit in the minimum time. They can be easily incorporated into even the busiest schedule, and represent a new and powerful tool to help keep you flexible, relaxed and in the best of health.

How to use this book

This book is divided into three parts.

The first part is devoted to Five Minute Massages for one person and focuses on the five areas of the body most prone to stress and tension: the head and face; the neck and shoulders; the arms and hands; the front and back; and the legs and feet.

Within each section are several five minute sequences which concentrate on one specific part of the body such as the scalp or the abdomen, which you can work with, releasing tension and increasing flexibility. Each sequence is complete by itself although you can, if you wish, link up sequences to form longer massages.

Another option would be to link up various or even all the sections so that you massage the whole body. There simply is no right or wrong way to use this book – just dip into it as and when you want and experiment. You can use the sequences for when you ache, when you're low on energy or even because you're curious.

The second part of the book is devoted to Five Minute Massages for two people. The sequences included in this section work with a whole area of the body and are much more general. Here you can share any skills you have learnt in the self-massage section, relaxing a partner and leaving him or her feeling positive. Even if you've never worked with anyone before, your partner will be sure to appreciate your efforts.

One major feature of this book is the inclusion of *Power Points*, which are of vital importance in Eastern massage. These are points on the surface of the skin where the energy that flows in channels called *meridians* can be stimulated.

According to Eastern medical theory, these meridians are connected to every part of your body from the top of your head to the tip of your toes, supplying each cell, nerve, muscle, bone, tissue and organ with energy. These meridians are usually called after the main organ they are associated with, so there is the kidney, gall bladder and liver meridians. Most meridians run down both sides of the body.

If there are no blockages in the meridians, energy can flow freely through the whole body, and this creates a state of health. However, if a meridian becomes blocked or imbalanced, perhaps because of stiff muscles, then this might lead to the person feeling a bit sluggish or falling ill. By simply applying finger pressure to a Power Point, a meridian can be stimulated to flow more freely. These Power Points can also be used to alleviate specific common ailments (see pages 94-95).

We hope that you enjoy using this book and that you get everyone around you involved and regularly experiencing the power and benefits of the Five Minute Massage. So explore, recharge your batteries and unwind!

The Five Minute Massage has been designed so that it is suitable for everyone.However, there are certain circumstances when massage should be temporarily avoided.
These are when you:

- are intoxicated
- are ill [1]
- have had any recent accidents or injuries [1]
- have had any recent surgery
- are taking any medication or seeing the doctor [1]
- have any cardiovascular and/or circulatory problems such as:

  - thrombosis
  - acute heart conditions
  - varicose veins

- have any open wounds, inflammations or sores

- are pregnant [2]

1. In these cases massage can sometimes be of benefit, although you or your partner must be the ultimate arbiter of whether to receive or not. For example, if you have a cold or are taking medication for a minor ailment, then massage may make you feel better, but may also help your cold or ailment clear up.

2. In this case Five Minute Massage can still be experienced, but there are certain Power Points that should not be used. These are clearly indicated throughout the book.

If working with a partner, please check with them that they have no conditions which would prevent them from receiving a Five Minute Massage. Furthermore, if any situation arises where you are in doubt about whether to massage, then consult your doctor.

Keeping

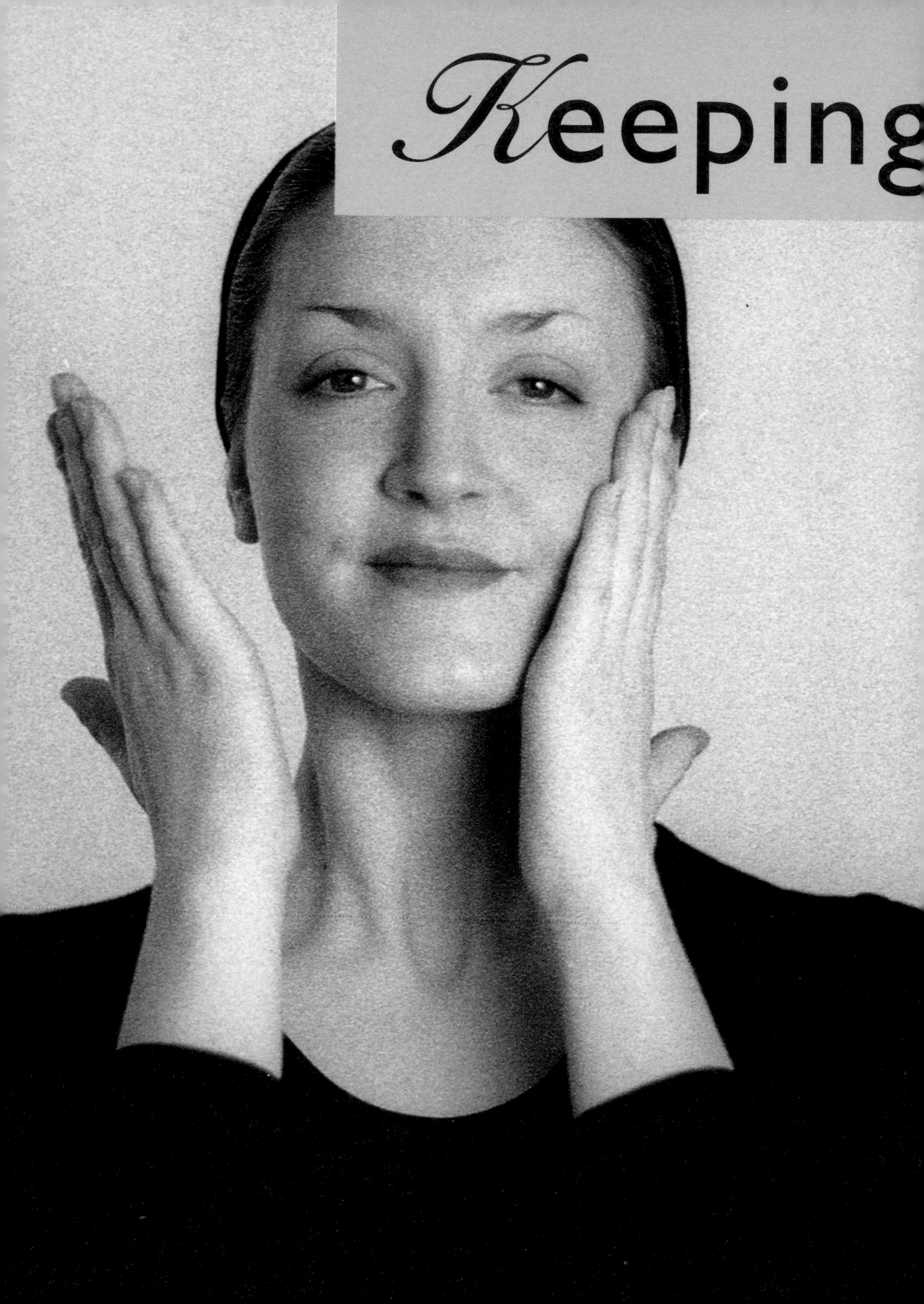

A Level Head

For most of us the head and face is the part of the body we are most aware of. This is because the main senses which gather information about the world around us – sight, hearing, smell and taste – are all located here.

The face is also the part of the body most on public display. It is a complicated and delicate structure in constant use, with dozens of small muscles acting in unison to create hundreds of expressions as we laugh, cry, talk or smile. Unfortunately, it is also the first place in the body where stress appears and can cause the scalp, eye, jaw and mouth regions to tighten which can result in a wide variety of ailments such as headaches, hair loss, eye strain, and neck and shoulder problems.

However, facial muscles which are subject to continual stress and tension exact an even higher price than the occasional headache – they are a principal cause of premature ageing as the muscles lose their elasticity, the skin loses its tone and wrinkles start to multiply.

Including a regular Five Minute Massage into your daily routine, particularly before you go to bed, is a simple and natural way of reducing stress and tension, as well as taking years off you.

So go on. Forget headache pills and anti-wrinkle creams. The key to feeling relaxed, young and vibrantly alive lies in your talented fingers. In today's busy world there's no better way to balance body and soul, and help you keep a level head.

*B*ecause it's not a region that we often touch, the scalp can become tense without us realizing. A tight scalp can restrict the blood flow to the hair roots and starve them of vital nutrients, making them fragile and lacklustre. In addition, since the scalp connects the face and the back of the skull, tension here can restrict both these regions and can be a main factor in triggering headaches and migraines. Massaging the scalp, therefore, can help relax and loosen the whole area, increase circulation, strengthen hair roots, improve hair quality, relieve headaches and simultaneously calm mind and body.

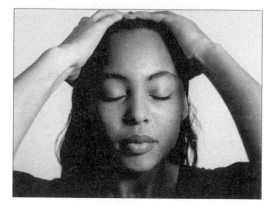

1 Begin by spreading your fingers at the top of the forehead and then slowly running them through your hair. This feels luxurious so spend a few moments enjoying it.

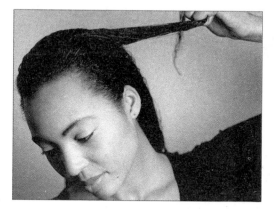

4 Run your fingers through your hair again, but this time stop in one place and gently grasp a handful of hair and give it a tiny tug. Rather than doing any damage, this move can actually strengthen the roots and also feels quite pleasant.

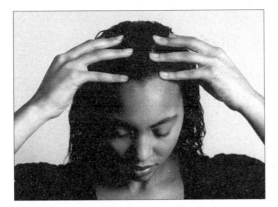

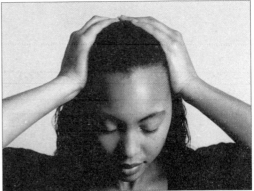

2 Then place the pads of your fingers on your scalp and begin to move them firmly in small circles, releasing the flesh underneath. Draw a couple of circles in one area and then move the pads to another place, searching for any tender spots. It is surprising how tight the scalp can become and just how good massage here can feel.

3 After your initial exploration with your fingers, use your palms to massage larger areas and apply deeper pressure. Be sure to use them to gently press the sides of the skull, and gently rotate.

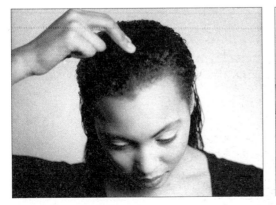

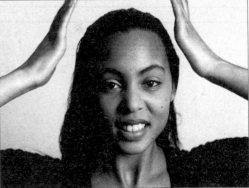

5 Then locate Governing Vessel 20 (GV 20) which lies at the top of the head, in line with the nose and between the ears. This point is good for boosting energy, relieving headaches and improving concentration.

NB: Do not use this point if you have high blood pressure.

6 As a finale, you can use the tips of your fingers to drum a gentle tattoo all over your scalp. This encourages blood flow to the region, and is very stimulating and energizing for the whole body.

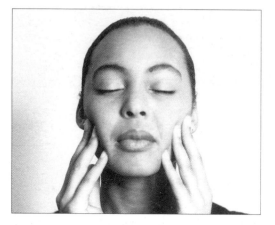

*S*ince we see our face reflected in the mirror every day, it would be natural to suppose that it would be the part of our bodies we'd be most familiar with. However, although we can instantly recognize ourselves, we rarely touch our own faces and so often remain unaware of the tension that lies hidden deep within our facial muscles. This sequence has been designed to reintroduce you to your face and will counteract the ageing process caused by tense facial muscles.

I Begin by gently rubbing your whole face with your fingertips. This loosens up the muscles and stimulates circulation. Next let your fingers explore the whole area, discovering if there are any tension spots.

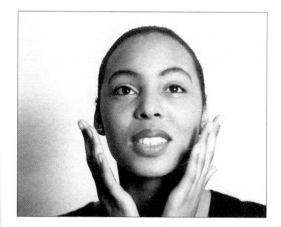

2 Then spend a few moments gently patting your face with your fingers. This really wakes the face up and brings tone and colour back to your cheeks.

3 Next you can have some fun by scrunching your facial muscles to pull various faces which will help loosen the area further. Experiment and see how many different faces you can pull. Can you do a bemused face, a gleeful face, a quizzical face, a frustrated face, a mean face? If you smile a lot, try some gruff expressions and discover how that feels. If you are generally serious, try some playful, silly expressions and see if you can make yourself laugh.

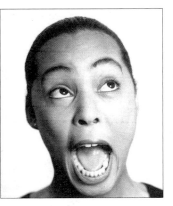

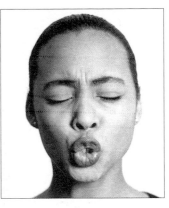

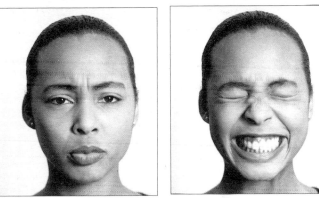

4 After really waking the face up, spend some time gently caressing it with your fingers. Start from the forehead and work your way down to the chin using nice long strokes which will help calm the area down and leave your face feeling relaxed and fully alive.

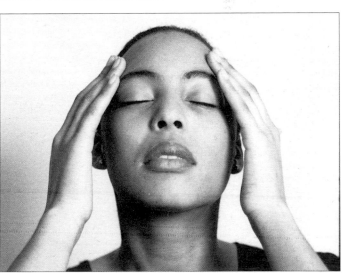

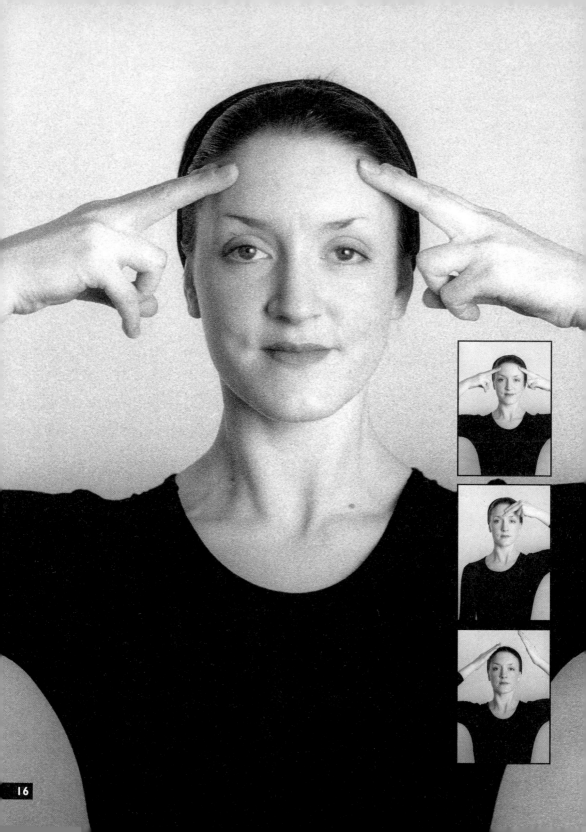

*W*hen we are troubled or making an effort to concentrate, our forehead and temples can often become tense and congested. Indeed, over time many people develop worry lines, which age them considerably.

This sequence is designed to help you to release tension, increase circulation, prevent and relieve headaches, and leave you feeling calm and looking younger.

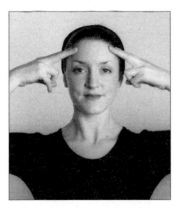

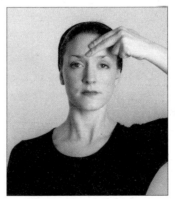

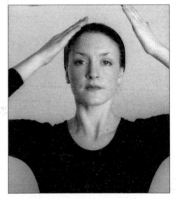

1 Put the tips of your fingers together and place them so that they are facing each other in the middle of the forehead. Gently bring them apart, fanning and smoothing the forehead in the process. Return to the centre and repeat five times. Then use the pads of your fingers to massage the forehead, starting at the top. Massage in small circles and work across the forehead in strips.

2 Using the first two fingers, press firmly between the eyebrows in line with the nose. This stimulates the Yintang point which is good for dispersing tension in the whole region.

3 End by gently patting the forehead and temple regions. This should leave you feeling energized.

The eyes are delicate structures, capable of focusing with pin-point accuracy on any object in our visual field. However, the muscles that move the eyeball to allow this are very rarely used to their full potential. Instead, most of us tend to lock our eye muscles, staring directly ahead for hours on end.

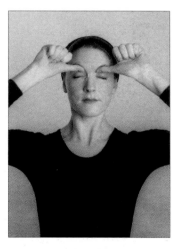

▌ Use the thumbs to press directly on the bone ridge at the rim of the eye socket. This point is Bladder 2 (B 2) and is good for releasing tension.

This tendency to stare for long periods is made worse by working with computers or watching TV. These can be very hypnotic and discourage you from using your eyes fully and can easily result in eyestrain, general fatigue and severe headaches. Massaging the eye region regularly, particularly while you work, can ensure that your eyes don't lose their movement capacity, and remain relaxed and in optimum condition.

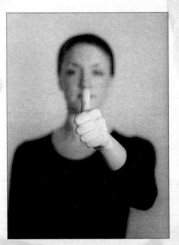

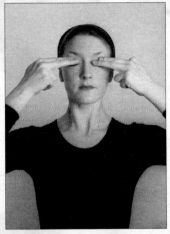

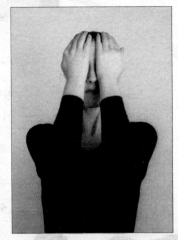

2 Place your thumb about 10 cm in front of you, then look at the tip of your nose, then at your thumb and then at something further away and then back to the thumb and nose again.

3 Close your eyes and slowly place the pads of your fingers on the eyelids. Then with the gentlest of pressure, massage the eyeball using small circles.

4 After these exercises, shut your eyes and cover them with the palms of your hands, allowing time to enjoy the darkness and warmth for a few moments. This helps release tiredness in the eyes and gives them a chance to rest. Slowly take your hands away, open your eyes and enjoy the difference.

*O*ne of the banes of modern life is the amount of pollution we all have to deal with. This can cause congestion, sinusitis and various breathing problems, which can affect how we feel and sap our energy. Massaging the nose and cheeks can keep nasal passages and sinuses free of congestion, and help ensure that you continue to breathe easily.

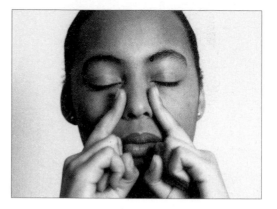

I Use two fingers to rub along the side of the nose. This can help clear and stimulate the sinuses. Then halfway down either side of the bridge of the nose is a point called *Bitong* which can help clear the nasal passages if pressed.

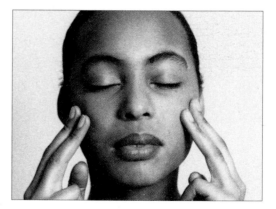

4 Loosen any tension and increase circulation to the area by using first your fingers and then your palms to move the cheeks in small circles.

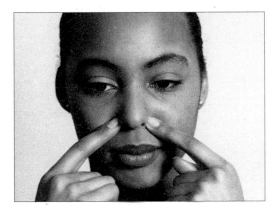

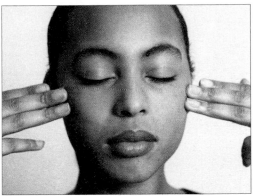

2 Then use your index fingers to press into the outside corner of each nostril where there should be a slight hollow. This is Large Intestine 20 (LI 20), also known poetically as *Welcome Fragrance*, which is good for rapidly clearing nasal and sinus congestion.

3 Next place your fingers flat on both cheeks and begin to pull them gently towards the ears. Then place your thumbs at the bottom of the cheeks, press inwards gently and trace their outline.

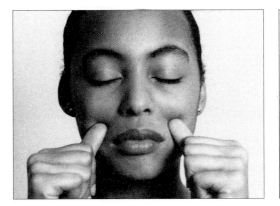

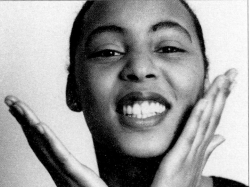

5 At the bottom of each cheek, directly underneath the pupil of the eye, is a little hollow which contains the point, Stomach 3 (ST 3). Pressing here can help to disperse tension, facial pain and general nasal congestion.

6 Rub your cheeks up and down with the fingers and then finish by gently slapping them to increase circulation and energy.

*A*lthough they are one of the most sensitive parts of our anatomy, the ears are a part of our body that we pay little attention to. Our hearing is one sense that never stops working even when we are asleep. So go on, give your ears a chance for some peace and quiet — give them a massage — you'll be surprised at how relaxing and calming this can be.

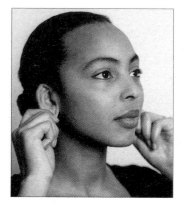

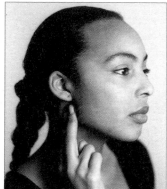

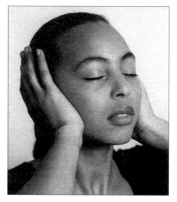

1 Begin by grasping both ears by the lobes and gently tug downward. Release and repeat working your way up the ear, pulling outwards and finally upwards. Then massage the whole area thoroughly by rubbing it gently between the thumb and the first finger.

2 Behind the ear are lots of points that are good for releasing tension and headaches. Work from the top of the ear to the bottom.

3 Finally, cover both ears with your hands and spend a few moments enjoying the sensation and quiet. At the end your ears should feel warm and tingly.

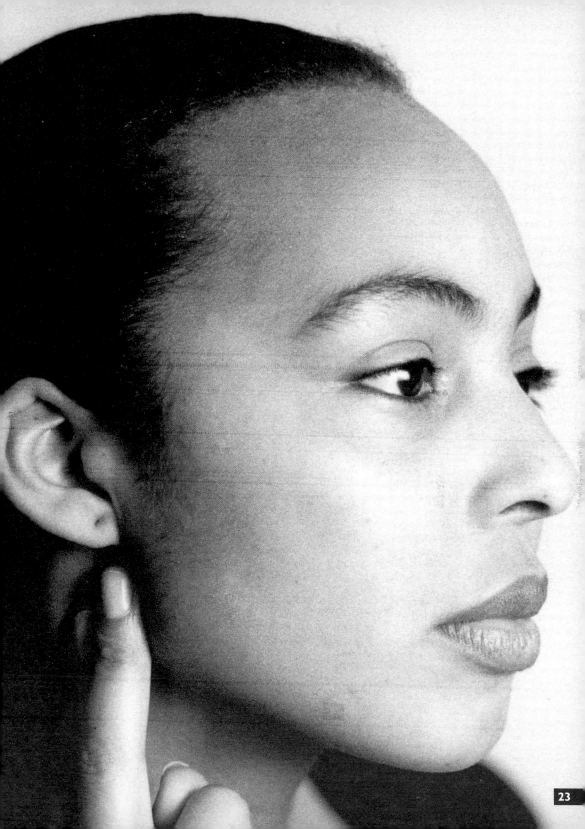

*I*n order to keep our jaws from uncontrollably falling open when we least expect it, our jaw muscles are designed to be contracted normally. The force involved in keeping these muscles constantly closed has been estimated by some experts to be around 242 kilos.

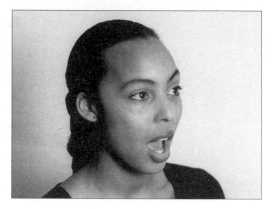

I Allow your jaw to descend gently and hang loose. Let it remain open for 10 seconds and then slowly close. Repeat this four times, allowing the jaw to open and drop further each time.

Excessive tension in this region can not only create sore jaw muscles, but because of the way the jaw connects with the rest of the skull can also be a major cause of headaches as well as hearing and visual problems. By directly massaging this area we can not only relieve tight jaws but also reduce overall facial tension.

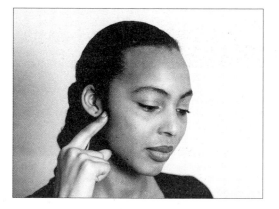

4 Gall Bladder 2 (GB 2) is found in the depression at the bottom of the ear. This may be a tender point to press, but is excellent for releasing jaw tension in addition to helping relieve toothache.

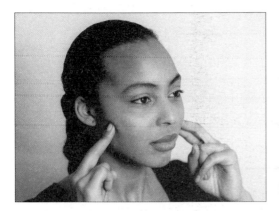

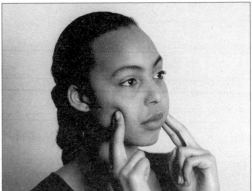

2 Now clench your teeth together. This makes the jaw muscles stand out, making them easier to locate. With the pads of your fingers press and massage these muscles in small circles. See if you can detect the muscles gently softening under your fingertips. If you want, you can use your palms as well to give the region a deeper massage.

3 Place the fingertips on the jaw muscles and then begin to gently drag them downwards towards the corners of the mouth. This helps to decompress the region and can often relieve pressure in the head. This will almost certainly feel tender, but worth doing for the benefits it brings.

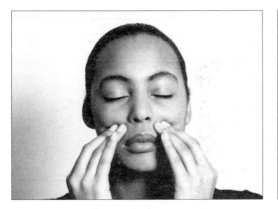

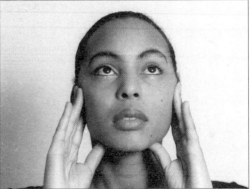

5 Then use all your fingers to relieve tension in the muscles around the mouth; this stimulates the gums at the same time.

6 Place your fingertips along the ridge of your jawbones on either side of your chin. Then place your thumbs underneath the chin, and press along the jaw bone with the fingers. This stimulates the salivary glands and reduces tension. After this gently press your thumbs along the underside of the jaw.

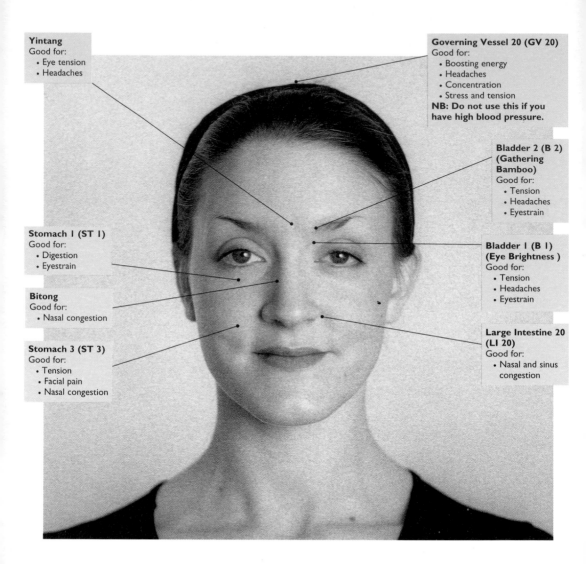

Yintang
Good for:
- Eye tension
- Headaches

Governing Vessel 20 (GV 20)
Good for:
- Boosting energy
- Headaches
- Concentration
- Stress and tension

NB: Do not use this if you have high blood pressure.

Bladder 2 (B 2) (Gathering Bamboo)
Good for:
- Tension
- Headaches
- Eyestrain

Stomach 1 (ST 1)
Good for:
- Digestion
- Eyestrain

Bitong
Good for:
- Nasal congestion

Stomach 3 (ST 3)
Good for:
- Tension
- Facial pain
- Nasal congestion

Bladder 1 (B 1) (Eye Brightness)
Good for:
- Tension
- Headaches
- Eyestrain

Large Intestine 20 (LI 20)
Good for:
- Nasal and sinus congestion

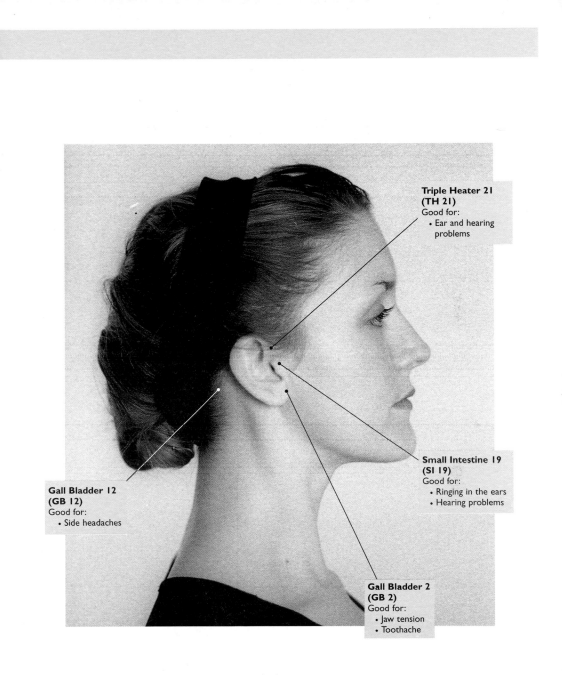

**Triple Heater 21
(TH 21)**
Good for:
• Ear and hearing
  problems

**Small Intestine 19
(SI 19):**
Good for:
• Ringing in the ears
• Hearing problems

**Gall Bladder 12
(GB 12)**
Good for:
• Side headaches

**Gall Bladder 2
(GB 2):**
Good for:
• Jaw tension
• Toothache

A Weight

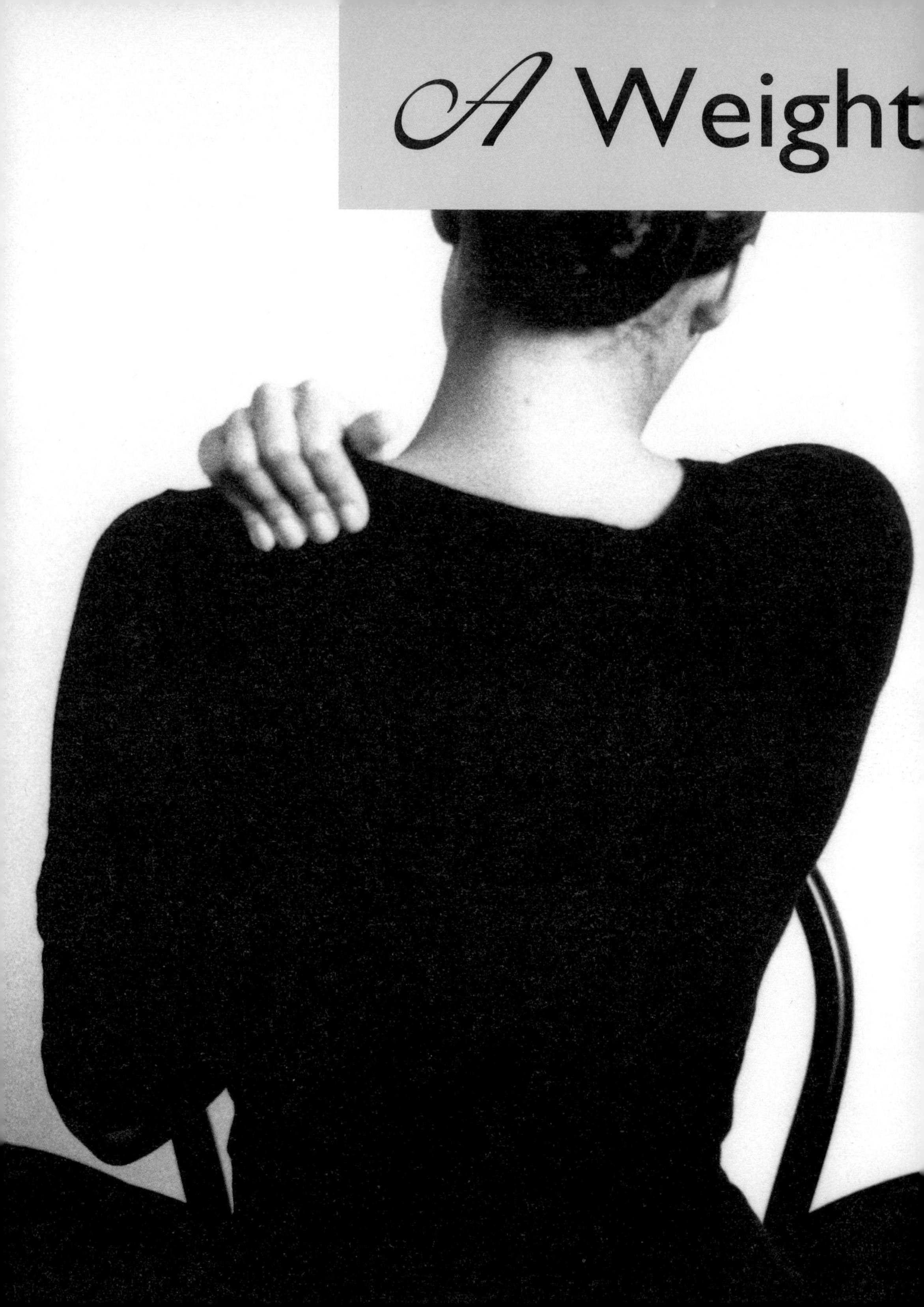

Off Our Shoulders

*R*are is the person who has never experienced any problems with their neck and shoulders: for most people it is the number one tension zone.

In its normal state, the head is designed to balance perfectly upon the neck vertebrae without imposing any strain. However, many of us tend to stick our necks forward a little when we're talking, concentrating or watching TV, and this throws our whole head out of alignment, resulting in the neck muscles having to tense up to take the full weight of the head, which weighs the equivalent of about six bags of sugar, or 5–7 kilos. A vicious spiral is then created where the muscles are constantly compensating for an unbalanced head, and end up permanently contracted, causing tremendous congestion and tightness, reducing neck mobility, and often resulting in headaches and eyestrain.

In addition, if the neck becomes tight, it can have a knock-on effect on the shoulders. A combination of a lack of movement caused by sitting for long periods and bad posture can lead to the shoulders slowly stiffening up and losing their flexibility. This has an immediate effect: restricting the ribs and how deeply we breath, slowing down the circulation, creating headaches and poor digestion, as well as tensing the entire body and throwing it out of balance.

Spending a few minutes every day massaging this region can help to loosen it up, release trapped energy and really take a weight off your shoulders.

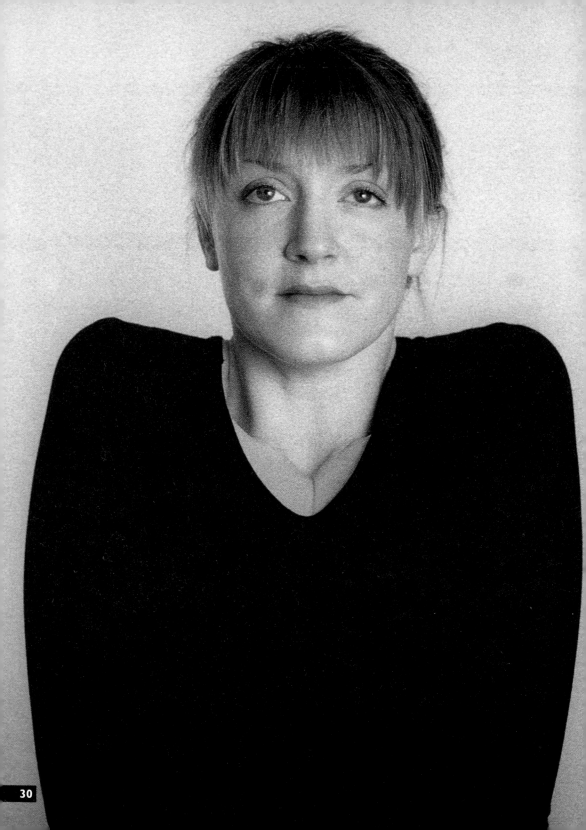

*W*alk down any busy street and chances are that most of the people around you will have their shoulders raised to their ears. Just why this is so, is a bit of a mystery, but discovering that our shoulders are keeping our ears company is quite a common experience. We might be surprised to find them there, and consciously make an effort to relax and allow them to drop, but within half an hour they've often stealthily crept back up again. This sequence will help you become aware of how you hold your shoulders, loosen the whole area, and bring them back down to where they should be.

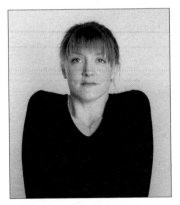

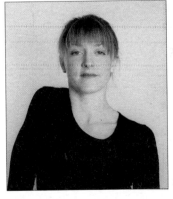

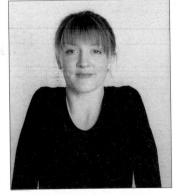

1 Take a deep breath and slowly raise your shoulders up to your ears as high as they can go. Then release them so that they fall back to their original position. Breathe out as you do so, and imagine that you are breathing out all the tension in that area. Repeat this three times.

2 Next begin to draw a circle with your right shoulder. Keep the circle small at first, and then slowly begin to create a larger circle with your shoulder, allowing the whole area to move freely. When you are ready, change direction and then repeat with the left shoulder.

3 Now that both sides have been warmed up, try moving your shoulders together in the same direction and draw different sized circles. Experiment. Can you feel any difference?

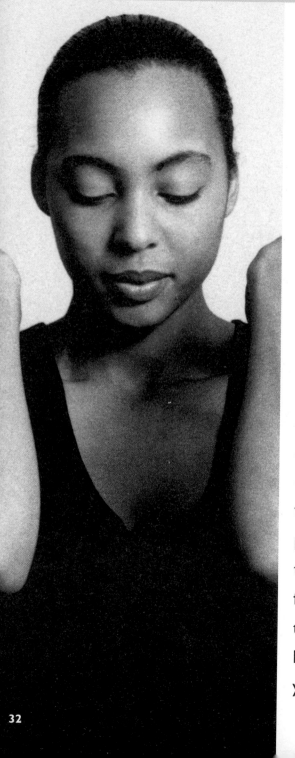

The shoulders are a very accurate barometer of our ability to flow and express ourselves freely. If they have slowly become tight and immobile throughout the years, then we may also find that we are beginning to lose our sense of spontaneity and adventure.

Releasing your shoulders can also release your ability to express your ambitions and feelings freely, allowing you to plunge into life, rather than tip-toeing around the edges. The following exercises will help you to loosen the whole region and let your energy flow. Express yourself.

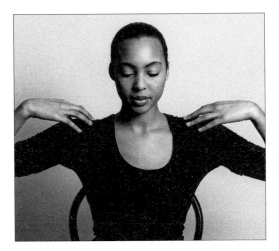

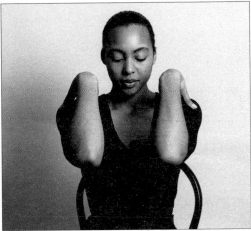

1 Rest your hands on each shoulder, and then begin to draw circles with your elbows, becoming aware of how the muscles move underneath your fingertips. Slowly allow the circles to get bigger, and observe how this affects the muscles. Change the direction and repeat.

2 With your hands still on your shoulders, slowly bring the elbows in as close together as you can. You should feel a good stretch in the middle of your back as you do this.

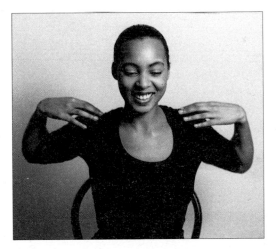

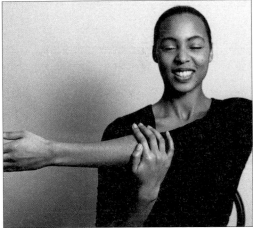

3 Take a deep breath and bring the elbows back as far as you can so that you can really open the chest area.

4 Stick your left arm straight out in front of you, and then with the right hand slowly pull the straight arm in towards the chest. You should feel the shoulder and upper back gently open up as you do so. Maintain the stretch for several seconds and then release slowly.

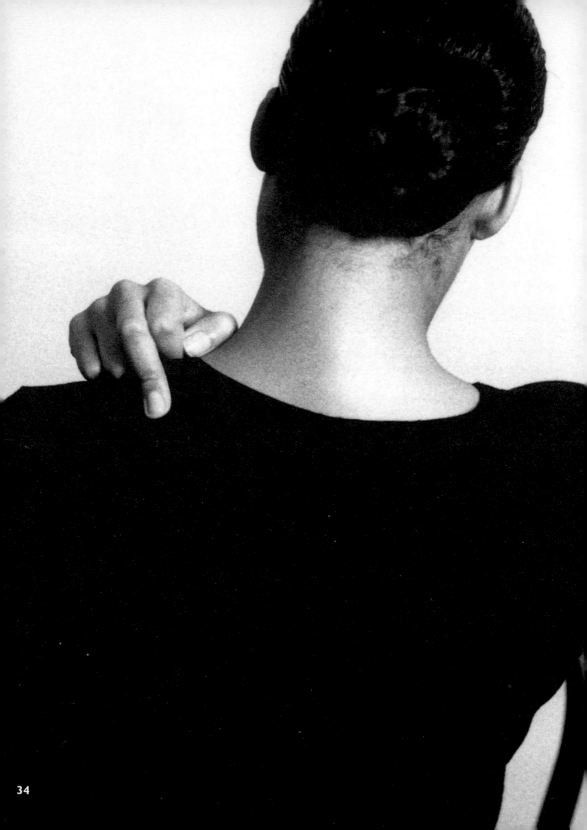

𝒯he more responsibilities we have – be they from work, looking after a family or just generally sorting our lives out – the more likely we'll begin to feel that 'I'm-so-burdened' feeling which often translates into a state of tension in the shoulders. The expression 'to shoulder responsibility' is not just a throwaway phrase then, but actually reflects a physical reality, which can really weigh us down and often feel oppressive. You can lighten the burden by trying this massage sequence.

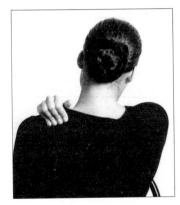 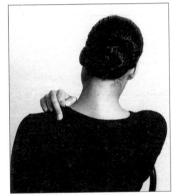 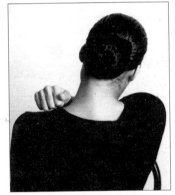

I Supporting your right elbow with your left hand, place your right hand on the top of your left shoulder and feel the muscle that runs from the top of the shoulder along the neck up to the back of the skull. Press into the muscle with the finger tips and begin to explore. Is it soft and pliable, or is hard, tough, tender even? What are your fingers telling you? Continue loosening the muscles in this area until you can detect the muscles softening up.

2 In the middle of the top of the shoulder, between the end of the shoulder and the base of the neck is Gall Bladder 21 (GB 21). This indicates mental stress and physical tension within the body, and is often tender to press. Stimulating it will help to release tightness in both mind and body.

Note: Do not stimulate if you are trying to conceive or are pregnant.

3 As a final shoulder technique, curl your hand into a loose fist, and softly begin to pound the area which has just been worked on. This will further loosen the muscles and also increase circulation in the area.

As anyone who has slept in a draught can confirm, a stiff or immobilized neck can not only be painful and uncomfortable, but also highlights how much we use our neck in daily life, and to what extent we depend upon it to remain flexible and unrestricted.

Sticking our chin out slightly can lead to the head becoming unbalanced with one set of neck muscles becoming over-constricted, while the opposite set becomes weakened, often resulting in headaches, eyestrain, and even neck vertebrae being displaced.

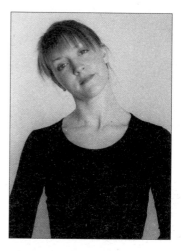

Keeping your shoulders by your side, gently tilt your head towards the right shoulder, feeling the stretch on the opposite side as you do so. Then repeat on the left side and bring your head back to the centre.

It is worth regularly spending some time on the neck area, releasing stored tension, balancing the neck and making sure it remains in good shape.

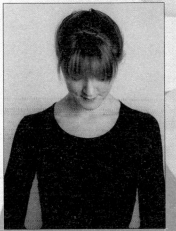

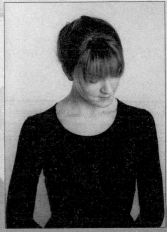

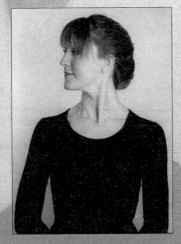

2 Now allow your head to fall forward gently. This allows the muscles at the back of the neck to lengthen and stretch. Bring your head back slowly and repeat twice more, each time allowing the weight of your head to increase the stretch a little further, if possible.

3 This is similar to the preceding move, but instead of looking straight down, look slightly to the left. As your head moves down, you should feel the back of your neck and the muscles in your shoulders being stretched.

4 Turn your head slowly to look to your right. Return to the centre and then continue moving your head to look over to your left. Repeat several times, each time trying to look a little further right and left, without straining.

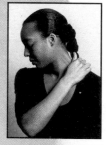

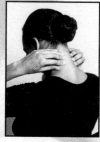

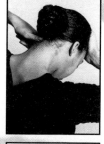

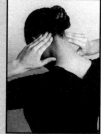

𝒯he neck is designed to be highly mobile. However, as we get older, our neck muscles can become tense and stiff, and it can become more difficult to move our head freely.

In addition, tension in this region can often cause surrounding areas such as the shoulders, upper back and chest to stiffen in turn. Regularly spending a few minutes massaging your neck can help to ensure that it remains relaxed and flexible.

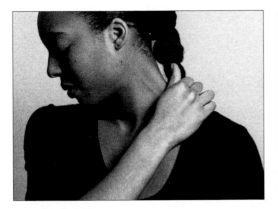

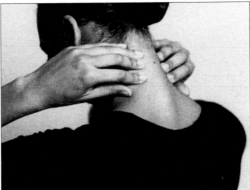

1 First tilt your head slightly to the right. This stretches the neck muscles on the left hand side. Now place your right hand on the side being stretched, and begin to massage the area using the palm and fingers in a kneading motion. Work the area well, and then change sides.

2 Then place your fingertips so that they are facing each other on either side of the neck, and begin to vibrate the muscles. Move progressively outwards, again searching for areas of tension.

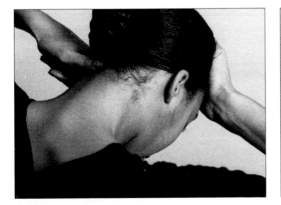

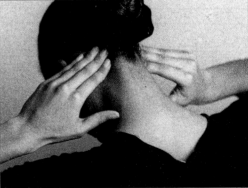

3 Support your forehead with one hand and place the thumb of the other hand in the centre of the back of the skull, where you should feel a small hollow. Governing Vessel 16 (GV 16) is located here and a lot of tension around the back of the skull can be released by stimulating this point.

4 Lastly, use your fingertips to massage the muscles around the back of the skull, which are often very tight and constricted. Try using small circles as you massage.

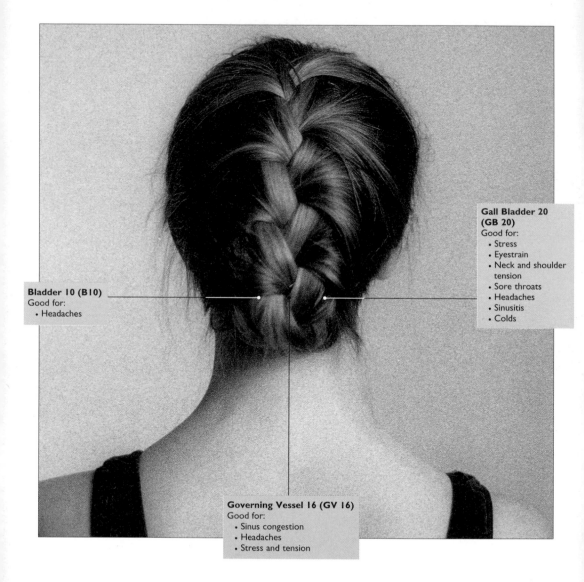

Gall Bladder 20 (GB 20)
Good for:
- Stress
- Eyestrain
- Neck and shoulder tension
- Sore throats
- Headaches
- Sinusitis
- Colds

Bladder 10 (B10)
Good for:
- Headaches

Governing Vessel 16 (GV 16)
Good for:
- Sinus congestion
- Headaches
- Stress and tension

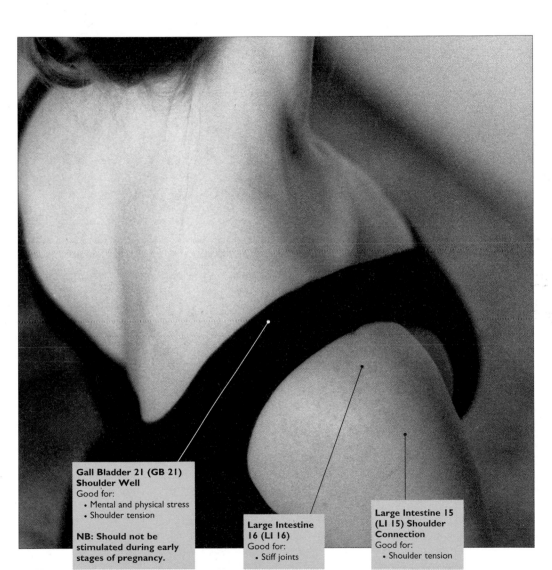

**Gall Bladder 21 (GB 21)
Shoulder Well**
Good for:
- Mental and physical stress
- Shoulder tension

**NB: Should not be
stimulated during early
stages of pregnancy.**

**Large Intestine
16 (LI 16)**
Good for:
- Stiff joints

**Large Intestine 15
(LI 15) Shoulder
Connection**
Good for:
- Shoulder tension

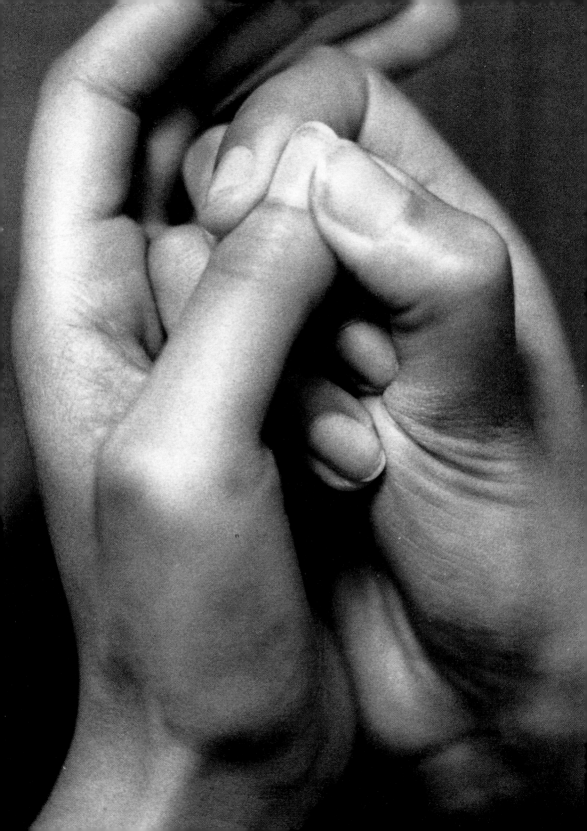

Hanging Loose

*E*ver since we first stood up on two feet, our arms and hands have been our chief tools in helping us shape and explore our environment. Through them we can perform hundreds of complex tasks and movements such as gripping, throwing, painting and writing. In addition, they also help us to express ourselves; to communicate our deepest emotions. Caressing and embracing, punching and shaking — these are all actions which let others experience our true feelings.

Our arms and hands are dynamic and expressive parts of our body, and are clearly very important to us. However, because they are in constant use, stress and tension can easily accumulate in the muscles and joints. Through time, it can begin to affect us, causing headaches and even pain in the neck, shoulders and back.

When you do these massages, you may be surprised to discover just how much tension your arms and hands hold. It is worth spending some time every day taking care of them and acknowledging how much work they do for you. Afterwards, you should feel as if they've been given a new lease of life — relaxed, energized and hanging loose.

*I*f you want to feel sorry for a part of your body, then feel sorry for your arms since they never have a chance to relax fully: they are always in a state of semi-tension. This is mainly because the upper arm muscles (the biceps and triceps) work as a pair and take turns to relax and contract.

So be kind to your arms and try the following massage, which will help them relax, banish stored tension and improve circulation.

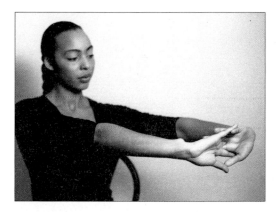

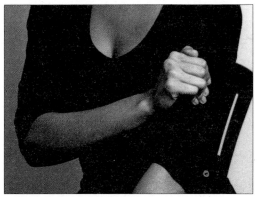

1 Interlock your hands, with the palms facing outwards and extend your arms in front. Keeping the arms straight, and the trunk as still as possible, swing them first to one side and then to the other and slowly bring them back to the centre. Finally raise your arms straight up and stretch and then return gently to your starting position.

2 Start with your right arm. Work all the muscles in the upper arm, squeezing each one between your thumb and fingers, and lifting it away from the bone. Then begin kneading, squeezing and rolling the muscles even more, exaggerating the movement.

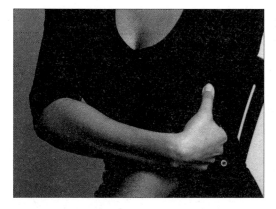

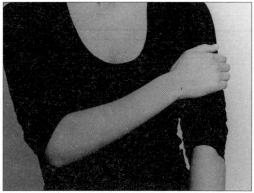

3 A useful Power Point to stimulate is Large Intestine 14 (LI 14) which is located at the bottom of the outside arm muscle (the deltoid). This is particularly good for relieving arm, neck and shoulder tension.

4 When you have finished, rub your arm vigorously. This creates a feeling of warmth, stimulates circulation and increases the flow of energy in the arms. How do you feel now? Now repeat steps 2-4 on the other arm.

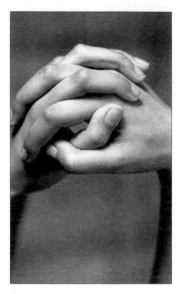

*W*hen you eat or drink anything that contains toxins harmful to the body, the body's response is to send all the toxins it can't eliminate to the joints in the limbs, keeping them as far away as possible from the vital organs in the centre. One joint that suffers particularly from this is the wrist, which can often become stiffer and stiffer. This is a delicate area full of tendons, nerves and blood vessels, and stiffness here can block the free flow of energy, and make it prone to inflammation or injury. Daily massage can ensure that the wrists remain supple and free of toxins, and ensure a free flow of energy throughout the whole arm.

I Interlock the fingers of both your hands and begin to trace a figure of eight with your hands. See how easily you can trace this figure, and whether there is any restriction of movement. Then change directions.

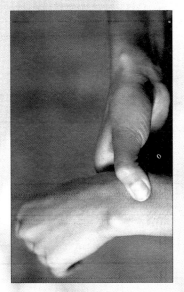 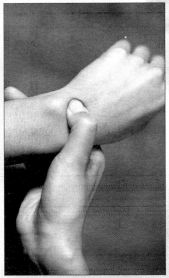 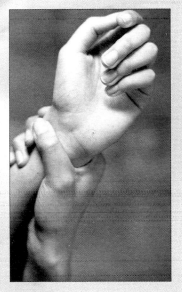

2 Then use the pads of your thumb to work around the area of the wrist, remembering to massage the back as well as the front of the wrist.

3 On the wrist crease on the back of the hand in line with the ring finger is Triple Heater 4 (TH 4). This is a very useful Power Point which can provide you with extra energy during the day, as well as relieving stiffness in the shoulder, arm, wrist, and increasing circulation in the hands. Support the hand as you press this point.

4 Hold the wrist with one hand. Gently squeeze and shake out fully. It should now feel more energized and relaxed.

HAND IN HAND

The hands are one of the most complex structures in our body: of the 30 bones in the whole arm, 27 are to be found in the hand, making it particularly susceptible to stress and tension. The good news is that they are exquisitely sensitive, and love being massaged. Doing so also stimulates several points in the hands which can help soothe and balance the rest of the body.

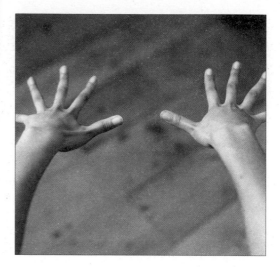

Make a fist with both hands and then slowly open your hands as much as possible so that the fingers are splayed out in a wide stretch. Repeat several times, feeling the hands open up a little further each time.

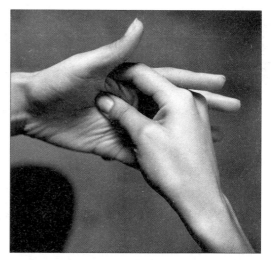

4 Interlock your fingers and turn the hands so that the palms are facing you. Now massage the palm of one hand with the thumb of the other. Use the thumb to move in small circles, gently massaging the whole of the palm.

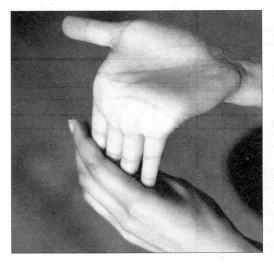

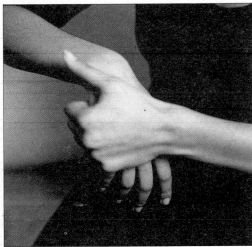

2 Take all the fingers of one hand and gently stretch them back. Then take the thumb and stretch that back.

3 Using your fingers as support, massage the back of the hand using your palm to cover the whole area. Then use the pad of your thumb to work the area in more detail.

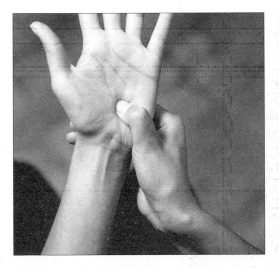

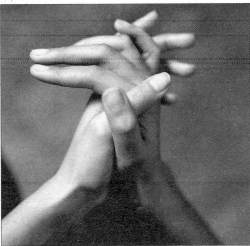

5 Called the *Palace of Exhaustion* in Chinese, Heart Governor 8 (HG 8) is a great pick-me-up point if you are tired, and is also good for stress and anxiety. This point is located where the ring finger touches the palm when it is bent. Now repeat steps 2-5 with the other hand.

6 Finally, gently rub both hands together as if you were washing them under a tap. This helps to increase the flow of blood and energy to the area. End by shaking both hands out thoroughly.

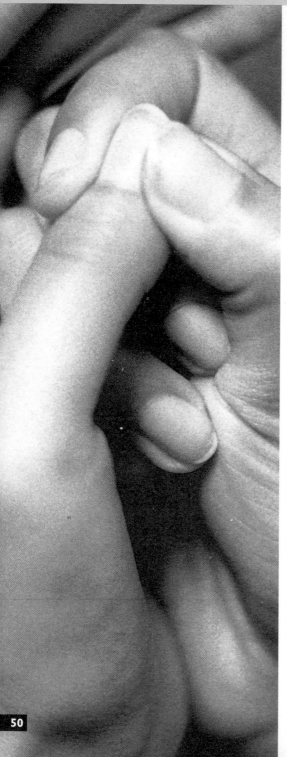

*O*ur fingers are constantly working for us, exploring the environment. In the process they often accumulate a lot of tension and frequently become less agile as we get older. To counteract this, regular finger massage will increase their flexibility and help keep them in great shape!

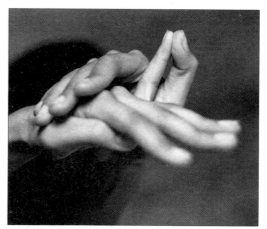

With the fingers of one hand supporting the back of the other, place the thumb at the base of the little finger and slowly push it along the finger so that the finger stretches back. Repeat with the other fingers.

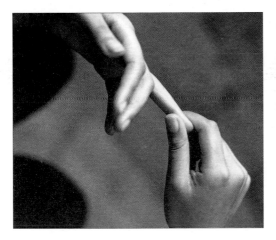

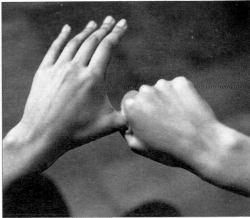

2 Take the little finger and begin to loosen it up by gently shaking it. Then start to rotate the finger in a clockwise direction. After a few moments, change directions and then continue with the remaining fingers.

3 Make a loose fist and slide your thumb inside. Close the fist to form a mini vice, and tug gently, which helps to loosen and lengthen the finger. Work the other fingers.

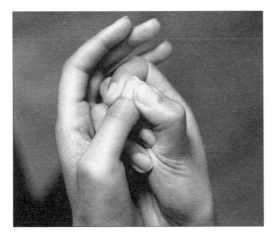

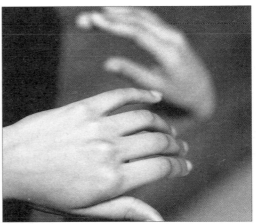

4 Squeezing each finger by the base of the nail can stimulate the flow of energy in the body. At the end of the thumb is Lung 11 (LU11), a particularly good point which can help clear congestion in lungs and sinuses, help sore throats and clear colds. Work all the fingers in the same way.

5 Finally, shake your hands out, and see how your fingers feel. They should feel lighter and perhaps even a little tingly.

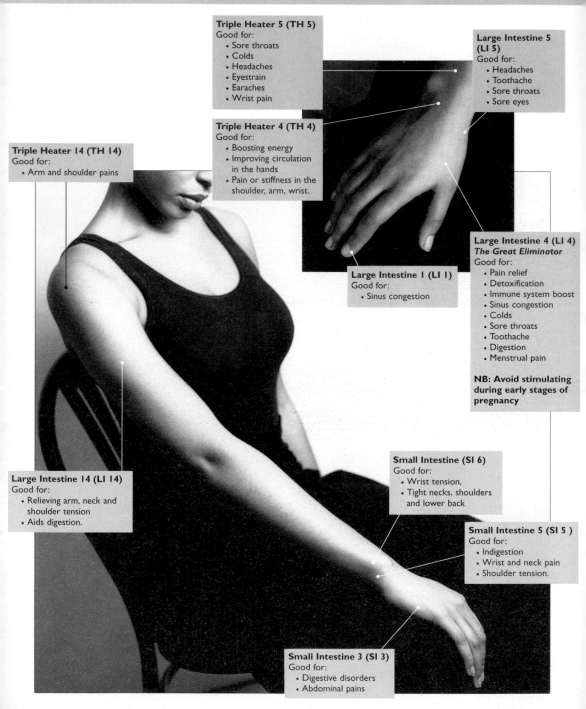

Triple Heater 5 (TH 5)
Good for:
- Sore throats
- Colds
- Headaches
- Eyestrain
- Earaches
- Wrist pain

Large Intestine 5 (LI 5)
Good for:
- Headaches
- Toothache
- Sore throats
- Sore eyes

Triple Heater 4 (TH 4)
Good for:
- Boosting energy
- Improving circulation in the hands
- Pain or stiffness in the shoulder, arm, wrist.

Triple Heater 14 (TH 14)
Good for:
- Arm and shoulder pains

Large Intestine 1 (LI 1)
Good for:
- Sinus congestion

Large Intestine 4 (LI 4)
The Great Eliminator
Good for:
- Pain relief
- Detoxification
- Immune system boost
- Sinus congestion
- Colds
- Sore throats
- Toothache
- Digestion
- Menstrual pain

NB: Avoid stimulating during early stages of pregnancy

Large Intestine 14 (LI 14)
Good for:
- Relieving arm, neck and shoulder tension
- Aids digestion.

Small Intestine (SI 6)
Good for:
- Wrist tension,
- Tight necks, shoulders and lower back

Small Intestine 5 (SI 5)
Good for:
- Indigestion
- Wrist and neck pain
- Shoulder tension.

Small Intestine 3 (SI 3)
Good for:
- Digestive disorders
- Abdominal pains

Lung 5 (LU 5)
Good for:
• Harsh, dry coughs

Heart 3 (H3)
Good for:
• Reducing stress
  and tension

Lung 4 (LU 4)
Good for:
• Colds
• Coughs
• Asthma and general
  breathing difficulties

Large Intestine 11 (LI 11)
Good for:
• Colds
• Sinus congestion
• Arm pain
• Stiff elbows
• Digestive problems
• Constipation

Large Intestine 10 (LI 10)
Good for:
• Stimulating circulation.

Heart Governor 6 (HG 6)
Good for:
• Travel sickness/nausea
• Indigestion
• PMS

Heart 7 (H 7)
Good for:
• Calming and relaxing an
  agitated mind
• Easing chest pain
• Palpitations

Heart Governor 7 (HG 7)
Good for:
• Travel sickness/nausea
• Anxiety

Heart Governor 8 (HG 8)
Palace of Exhaustion
Good for:
• Boosting energy
• Colds
• Chest pain
• Stress and anxiety

Lung 9 (LU 9)
Good for:
• Strengthening the lungs,
• Sinus congestion,
• Colds
• Athma
• Chest pain
• Sore throats

Lung 10 (LU 10)
Good for:
• Congestion in
  lungs and sinuses
• Colds
• Asthma

Lung 11 (LU 11)
Good for:
• Congestion in
  lungs and sinuses
• Sore throats
• Colds

Back By

Popular Demand

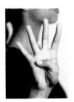

The back is a very strong part of our body, keeping us upright and preventing us from collapsing. It is composed of the spine – 33 vertebrae stacked on top of each other – and a complex lattice of muscles, which together permit a high degree of movement, mobility and flexibility. Yet this is also one of the regions most vulnerable to muscular tension, strain and traumas which can be debilitating and excruciating.

It is estimated that 75 % of the population or three out of every four people will have a problem with their back at some point in their lives. This may range from a nagging general ache to full-blown sciatica or even a slipped disc. However, in traditional societies the incidence of back pain and related problems is very low.

Whereas traditional peoples spend a lot of their time squatting close to the ground, we spend long periods sitting in chairs. Although lacking the sophistication of a chair, squatting is far healthier for the body since it opens and stretches the back muscles rather than subjecting them to unrelenting pressure and tension.

In addition, the back is often pushed to its limits as it tries to deal with a variety of other factors such as; soft beds, poor posture, carrying heavy bags and incorrect lifting techniques which can all take their toll and lead to a whole host of back problems through time.

Massage is one of the best ways to help counter some of these problems, since it relaxes and releases tight muscles, and increases flexibility and mobility. Taking five minutes regularly to work with the back can be one of the best investments you can make since it can help to diffuse a lot of the tension which builds up unnoticed and which can later wreak total havoc.

*T*he back is the major blind spot in our body, and since it is out of sight it is all too easy to lose awareness of this area. However, a lot of the tension that builds up on a day-to-day basis as we spend long hours hunched over a computer or at the steering wheel can be successfully dispersed if tackled regularly with massage.

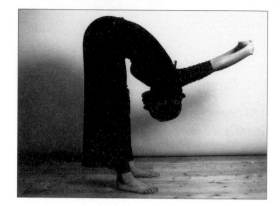

1 Stand with your feet apart and then lock your hands together behind your back. Slowly bend forward and let your head hang loose so that the arms gently start to rise. When you have gone as far as you can go, slowly bring them back down and come back into an upright position. This move not only stretches and loosens the upper back, it also works to stimulate several meridians.

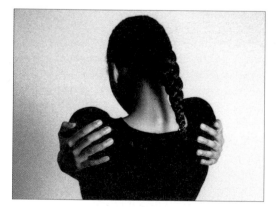

3 Cross your arms so that your left hand is grasping the right shoulder and vice versa. Then let the fingers of each hand walk towards the centre of the back. You should feel a good stretch there as your hands move closer towards each other, but don't worry if the hands don't meet.

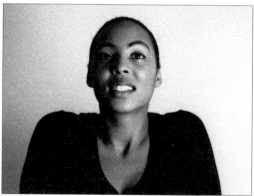

4 You can loosen the upper back further by rolling your shoulders in large circles. Really experiment and move your shoulders in different directions. The more you restore mobility to the region, the less opportunity there will be for tension to develop.

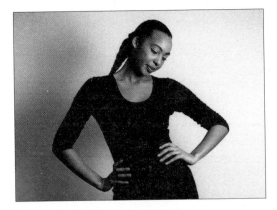

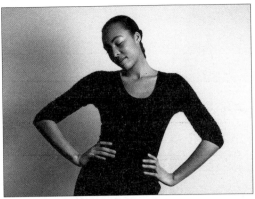

2 Next stand with your hands on your hips and gently begin to rotate from side to side.

This loosens your upper body and you may also hear a couple of clicks as various bones are realigned. Don't be too enthusiastic with this stretch. Gently does it.

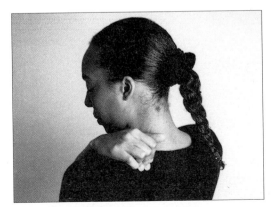

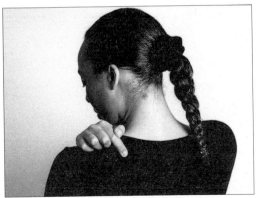

5 Begin to knead the tops of the shoulders, changing hands where necessary. Use your fingertips to locate any tight areas around the tops of the shoulders and the shoulder blades.

6 Then at the top corner of each shoulder blade, press into the little hollow located there. This will stimulate Small Intestine 14 (SI 14), one of the most effective points for relieving neck, shoulder and back tension. End your massage by gently brushing down the whole area.

The lower back is one of the high risk zones of the body. Long hours spent sitting in chairs day after day, year after year can cause compression of the vertebrae and a build-up of tension that can lead to a slipped disc and even sciatica. Sitting with your legs crossed can be especially bad for the lower back since it continually contracts one side while considerably weakening the other, making the whole area vulnerable to strain.

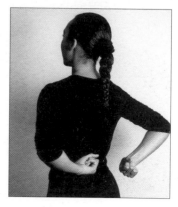

Warm up the lower back by making loose fists and gently striking the area. This stimulates circulation and helps to break up tension. Take care not to pound too hard around the kidneys which are located just below the bottom of the ribs.

Unfortunately, it is very easy to become used to the level of tension in this region because the process is so gradual; we think nothing of it until something goes drastically wrong. Regularly setting time aside to release and take care of your lower back will ensure it remains in optimum condition and that you don't have any unexpected setbacks.

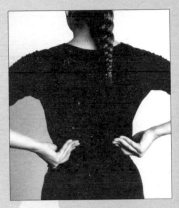 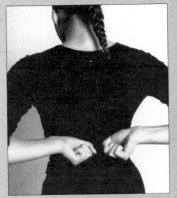 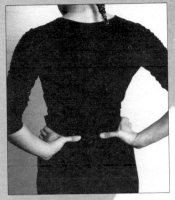

2 Slowly come back up and then use your fingers to explore the muscles running parallel to the spine. These are called the erector spinae and are largely responsible for keeping us upright, but they are especially prone to becoming tense through long periods of sitting.

3 Then work in small circles from the mid to the lower back using your fists or knuckles. If you place your hands on your hips, you can use your thumbs to pull the erector spinae slightly to one side and 'twang' them. This is a good way of releasing tight muscles.

4 Use your thumbs to press around the sacrum, which is a large bony area at the bottom of the spine. There are dozens of Power Points in this region which are especially good for relieving congestion, lower back pain and menstrual pain. Finally, calm and soothe the area with some gentle rubbing. How do you feel now?

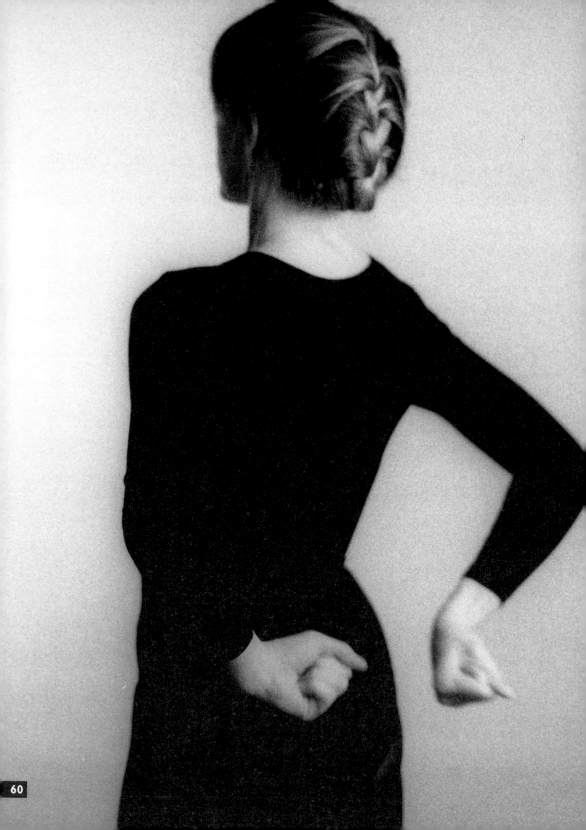

The pelvis is the bridge between the legs and the torso and helps to co-ordinate our movements. If we are tense or stiff in this region, then this can have a direct impact on the way we move and also affects our overall flexibility. It's a good idea, therefore, to ensure that the pelvis remains generally loose and supple. Furthermore, according to Oriental thinking, there is also a connection between the head and the bottom, so try pounding your bottom and see if your thinking becomes any clearer !

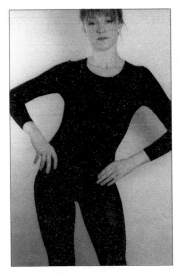
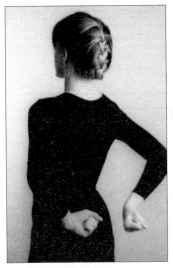
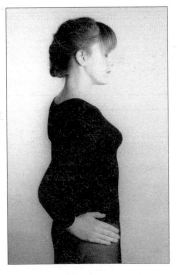

1 Place your hands on your hips and gently move the hips from side to side. Then begin to trace circles with your hips. Then begin to trace circles with your hips.

2 Then make a loose fist with both hands and begin to pound around the hips and buttocks. Don't pound too hard – just enough to get the blood flowing.

3 Finally, we are going to find and loosen any remaining tight muscles. Place the heel of one hand on the buttock muscles and massage the area in small circles. Be sure to explore the tops and sides of the whole region, not just the middle. Shake your hips and buttocks when you finish.

*O*ur most important organs, the heart and lungs, are housed in the chest. The heart is responsible for circulating blood and nutrients to every part of the body and the lungs are responsible for bringing in life-giving oxygen and expelling toxic carbon dioxide. These two delicate, vulnerable organs are protected by the ribs, which are a barrel-like structure circling the chest and back.

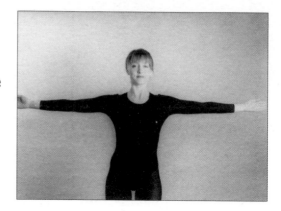

Begin by taking a slow, gentle deep breath, and open your arms wide as if preparing to embrace something large. This really expands and stretches the chest.

Tension in the chest can cause muscles to tighten in the shoulders, upper back and the ribs which can restrict breathing. Full relaxed breathing is important because it not only helps to oxygenize the blood but because it also massages the internal organs, improving the functioning of the lymphatic system, and helping to energize the whole body. Regular Five Minute Massage in this region can go a long way towards releasing accumulated tension and really get things off our chest.

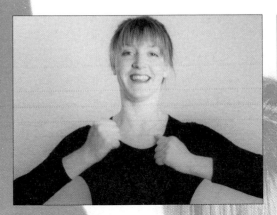

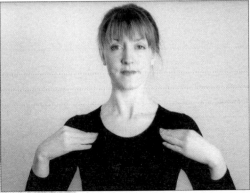

2 With a loose fist, begin to gently pound your chest, sides and abdomen, making Tarzan sounds, if appropriate. Pounding the chest like this boosts available energy, stimulates the immune system and strengthens the respiratory system.

3 Use the fingers of both hands to explore your pectoral muscles, which are just under your collarbone. See if you can find any tight spots, or areas that are a little tender. Spend some time massaging in small circles, or simply vibrating the fingers so that the area loosens up.

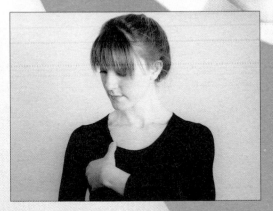

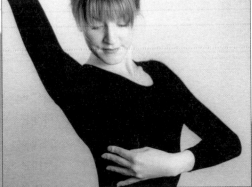

4 Next stimulate Lung 1 (LU 1) which is located an inch below the collar bone, next to the ribs. This is a useful point to work with since it can ease tight chests, acute coughs and asthma.

5 Finally, lift your arm and use the fingers or palms of your other arm to massage the side muscles. You can also use the fingertips to trace the ribs, vibrating the area to loosen them, but remember to keep breathing while you massage! Your chest should now feel considerably freer and relaxed.

*C*losely connected with our most basic drives – hunger and sex – the abdomen is the most exposed and vulnerable part of our body. It also houses our deepest intuitions or 'gut feelings', which can often reliably guide us to what is best for us. Unfortunately, in today's fast-moving world it is all too easy to ignore or mistrust the primitive wisdom of our raw emotions, and let our mind override their messages, often much to our cost.

Massage can help to readjust this imbalance, stimulating circulation, dispersing blockages and toxins, easing digestive and elimination problems and soothing muscular pains.

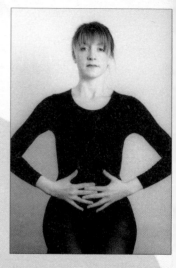

▌ Sitting down, place your hands on your abdomen and gently move them in a wide clockwise circle. Then work a little deeper with the tips of your fingers, creating mini-circles, yet still following a clockwise pattern. This massage softens tight abdominal muscles, helps digestion and can also ease constipation.

NB: If you are pre-menstrual or pregnant keep all the movements light and soothing.

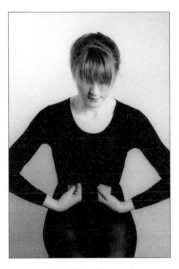

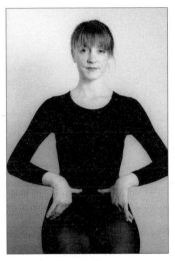

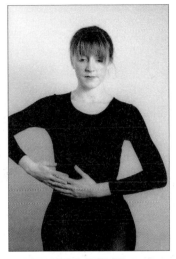

2 Place the fingers of both hands so that they are level with the bottom of one side of the rib cage. Slowly lean forward, allowing the fingers to sink into the area. If you gently push the fingers slightly up and make small circular movements, this will massage the internal organs. Repeat on the other side.

3 Next stimulate the Power Point Stomach 25 (ST 25). This is extremely good for increasing circulation in the bowel. It is located two thumb widths on either side of the navel.

4 Put the fingertips of both hands together so that they are touching each other and rest them on the abdomen. Now begin to rub the hands up and down lightly over the abdomen so that the movement creates some warmth. Slowly let your hands come to rest and begin a rocking movement from side to side, which will calm and soothe the area. Let this movement die away and spend some time with your hands just resting on your abdomen. Enjoy the sensation.

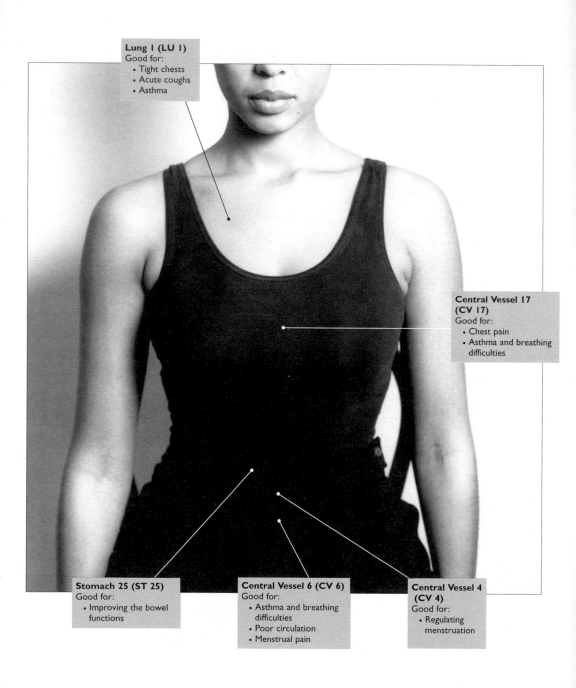

Lung I (LU I)
Good for:
- Tight chests
- Acute coughs
- Asthma

Central Vessel 17 (CV 17)
Good for:
- Chest pain
- Asthma and breathing difficulties

Stomach 25 (ST 25)
Good for:
- Improving the bowel functions

Central Vessel 6 (CV 6)
Good for:
- Asthma and breathing difficulties
- Poor circulation
- Menstrual pain

Central Vessel 4 (CV 4)
Good for:
- Regulating menstruation

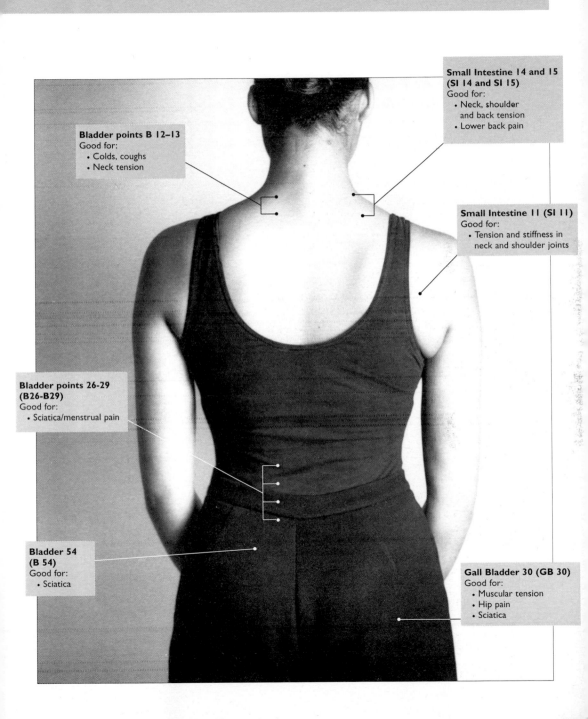

Small Intestine 14 and 15 (SI 14 and SI 15)
Good for:
- Neck, shoulder and back tension
- Lower back pain

Bladder points B 12–13
Good for:
- Colds, coughs
- Neck tension

Small Intestine 11 (SI 11)
Good for:
- Tension and stiffness in neck and shoulder joints

Bladder points 26-29 (B26-B29)
Good for:
- Sciatica/menstrual pain

Bladder 54 (B 54)
Good for:
- Sciatica

Gall Bladder 30 (GB 30)
Good for:
- Muscular tension
- Hip pain
- Sciatica

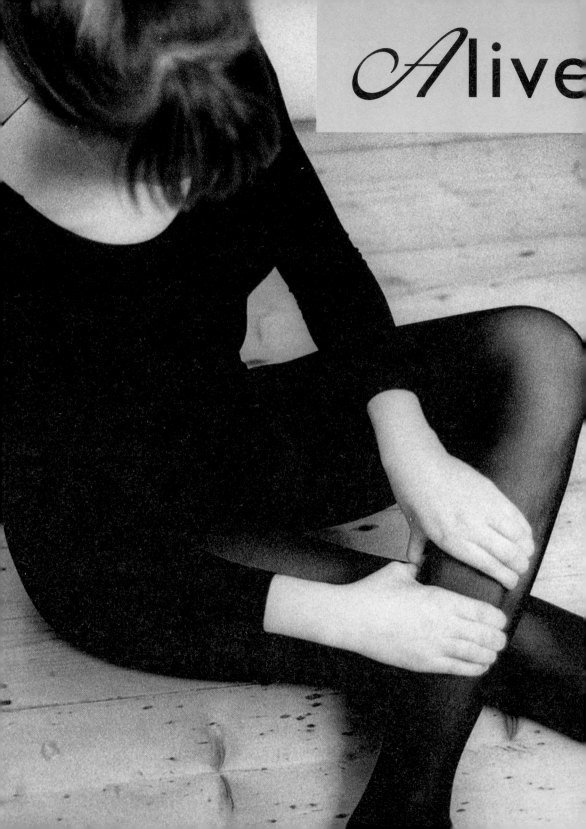

Alive

And Kicking

Our legs and feet are probably the hardest working and most neglected part of our body. Whereas our arms and hands are responsible for doing and expressing, our legs and feet are in charge of transporting us, for getting us from A to B.

With each stride dozens of muscles work together to provide a sturdy, steady platform, supporting our weight and providing us with stability. However, we often overlook this part of the body, trusting it to look after itself.

However, as with any part in constant use, the legs and feet are prone to becoming tense and tired, and if muscles become too stiff and tense they can begin to affect our free movement and even to sap our energy.

The feet are particularly prone to this, as they help to balance and support us, absorbing the shocks from walking and running. Unfortunately, tension can build up unnoticed and result in the feet losing their ability to provide good support and act as shock absorbers. Inevitably, this has a knock-on effect on the rest of the body, spreading tension to the ankles, knees, pelvis, lower back and spine.

Including a Five Minute Massage in your daily routine, particularly after you have been exercising or have been on your feet all day, is a simple and natural way of restoring life to your tired, aching legs and feet. So do yourself a favour: take a step in the right direction and get massaging. Five minutes is all it takes to leave you alive and kicking!

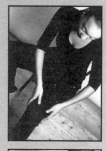

The thigh muscles are among the most powerful in the body, providing the momentum for walking, running and jumping. However, because a lot of our time is spent sitting down, our upper leg muscles often become contracted and tight through remaining in the same limited position. This stiffness blocks the free flow of energy throughout the leg, and can result in toxins building up. These simple and effective exercises will help keep your legs relaxed and free of harmful toxins as well as helping to reduce the bugbear of water retention and unwanted cellulite.

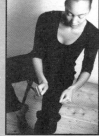

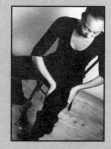

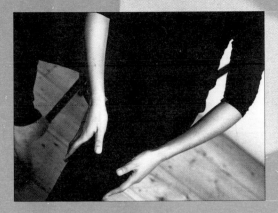

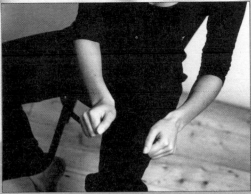

1 First take one leg and begin to gently stroke the whole leg right down to the foot. This will begin to loosen and relax the areas you will be working on.

2 Then with a loose fist pound the tops, side and bottom of the thigh and then the rest of the leg. This is a great pick-me-up if your legs are tired.

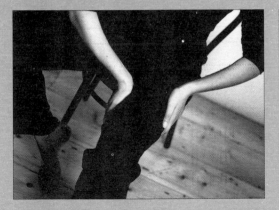

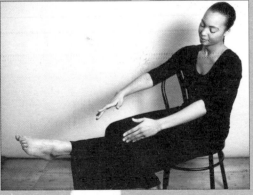

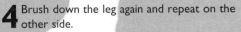

3 Next place your hands along the sides of the thigh and begin to shake and vibrate the muscles. Keep your hands loose and explore the region, using the heel of the hand for any tight spots.

4 Brush down the leg again and repeat on the other side.

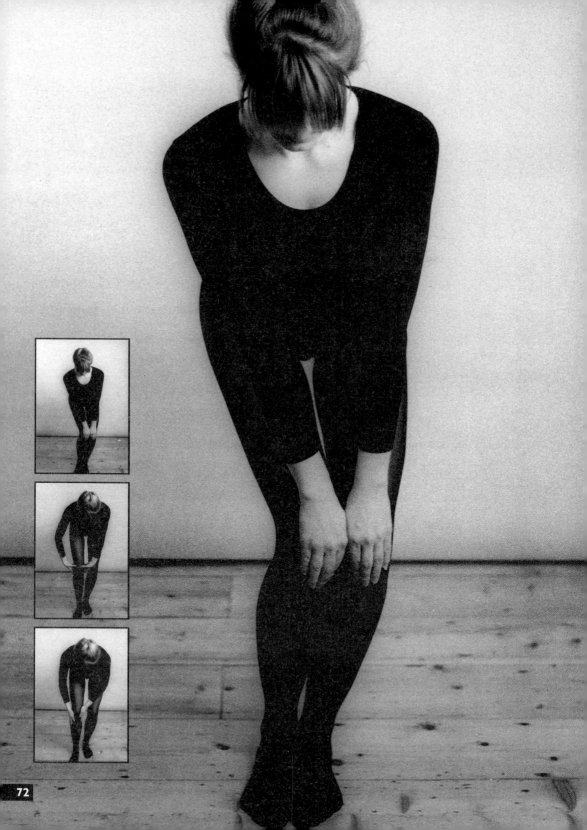

*Th*e knee is the largest joint in the body. It consists of the kneecap, and a lattice of protective muscles which provide great stability and also allow the legs a great deal of freedom of movement. However, the muscles which surround the knee joint can easily be compressed, exposing the joint to twisting, which can create stiffness and instability. Working here can help release any tension held and restore the knee to its full range of movement.

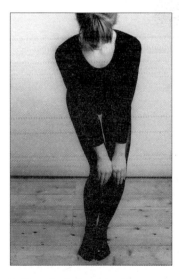

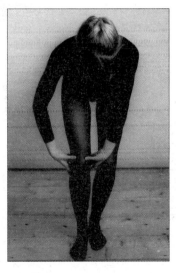

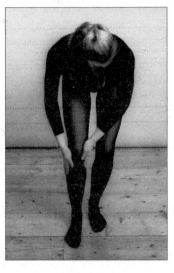

1 Place both feet together so that your knees are as close as possible. Then put your hands on your knees and imagine that there is a large pencil held between them. Now imagine you are drawing small circles on the ground with this big pencil by making tiny clockwise circles with your knees. This is a good exercise for releasing any stiffness in the joint.

2 Then place your two hands around the right knee and press all around the kneecap. The depressions just above and below the kneecap are particularly useful for easing knee joint stiffness and pain.

3 Next place your palms on either side of the knee and gently begin to vibrate the whole area. Switch to your fingertips and begin to massage the sides in small circles. Then do the same to your left knee.

*T*he lower legs take a lot of the strain of standing all day, and the impact every time we walk, run and jump. Not surprisingly, the calf muscles are often extremely tight, full of toxins, prone to cramps, and a prime target for varicose veins.

Massaging the lower legs can release stored tension, increase circulation and return them to full efficiency. Working here might be tender, but it's worth it to release the energy locked up in these tight muscles and restore the body. This sequence is best carried out sitting on the floor so that you can work with your legs easily.

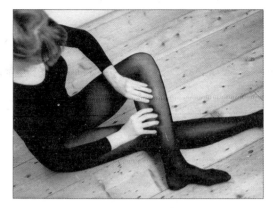

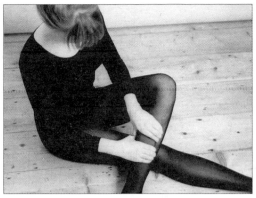

1 Sitting down on the floor, place your foot on your other leg and massage the calf as if you were kneading dough. If you find any tight or tender spots in the muscles, use your thumbs to zone in and loosen them.

2 If you place your two thumbs at the back of the calf, the fingers of the outside hand should be touching a band of muscle which runs alongside the shin bone. Use all your fingers to massage this muscle, which often gets very tight.

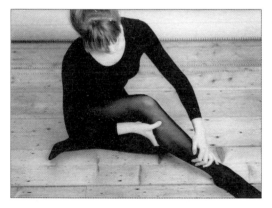

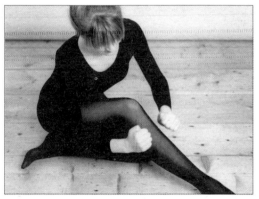

3 During the Long March of 1934 Chinese soldiers would stimulate Stomach 36 (ST 36) to help them with their punishing 6000-mile march. This point can be found four finger widths below the tip of the kneecap in the groove between the shin and outer bone. This point not only boosts energy within the body, but also relieves tired legs, headaches, and strengthens the immune system.

4 After working with the Power Points in the lower leg, spend a few moments gently vibrating and then pounding the calf muscles. Shake your leg out and repeat on the other side.

*A*s anyone who has had a sprained or twisted ankle can confirm, the ankle is a very important part of our body: a small, flexible region which connects the foot with the rest of the body, and acts as a shock absorber, supporting our entire weight.

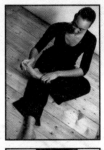

However, it is also very easy for tension to accumulate here, causing the ankles to stiffen, and become more susceptible to injury. Once this process begins, the free flow of energy between the feet and legs can be disrupted, and tension can begin to spread and cause problems in other parts of the body – the back, for example. Regular massage can help to prevent this.

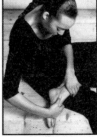

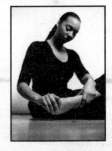

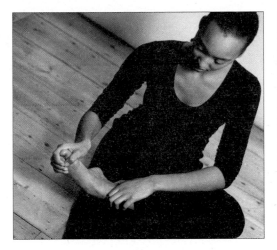

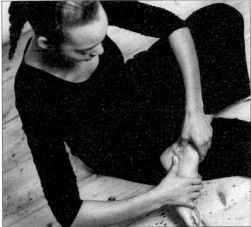

1 Sitting down on the floor, take one foot in your hands and begin to rotate the ankle. See if you can complete a smooth circle. If there are any restrictions, keep working the ankle and change direction when appropriate.

2 Then use your thumb to massage the whole ankle joint. Spend some more time on any areas that feel particularly tender or tight.

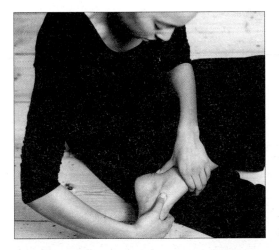

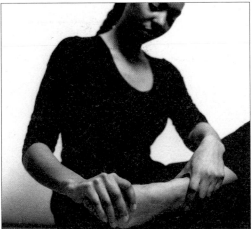

3 If you place your thumb just below the inside ankle bone and let your thumb slide a little towards the front of foot, you should find a little hollow. Spleen 5 (SP 5) is located here and can be stimulated to relieve tired and aching ankles. This point relieves tired, aching feet too!

4 Finally, stretch the foot downwards and then back upwards – this releases any remaining tension.

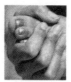 *N*o other part of the body is quite as abused, neglected or undervalued as the feet. They are highly complex structures: intricate webs of nerves, tendons, muscles and bone which are designed to provide a stable base to allow us to transfer our weight and move smoothly. Each foot contains 26 small bones and 32 joints, supporting our whole weight and absorbing the shock as we walk, run and jump, making the foot one of the strongest, most elastic and flexible parts of the body.

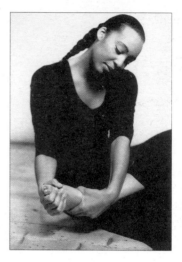

▌ Take a foot in both hands and work your way down, beginning at the top, wringing and twisting the bones along the foot. You can also begin to make larger movements, which will increase the overall flexibility of the area.

The feet work very hard for us and deserve to be taken care of. Regular massage will release stored tension, increase flexibility and circulation in the feet as well as help to relax, refresh and balance your whole body. Once you begin to take care of your feet, they will never forget how good massage feels, and they will always be there to take you one step beyond.

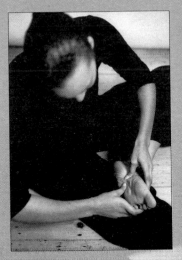

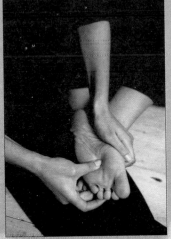

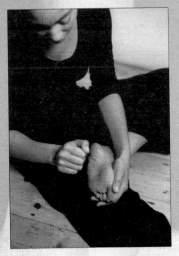

2 Now use both thumbs and your intuition to explore and massage the bottom of the foot, releasing any tight spots.

3 Next take hold of the little toe and gently rotate it. Continue with all the others, and then pinch and tug at the tip of each toe to stimulate the flow of energy throughout the foot.

4 After having thoroughly loosened and massaged the foot, pound it all over: this will stimulate the whole body. Shake out and repeat the sequence on the other foot.

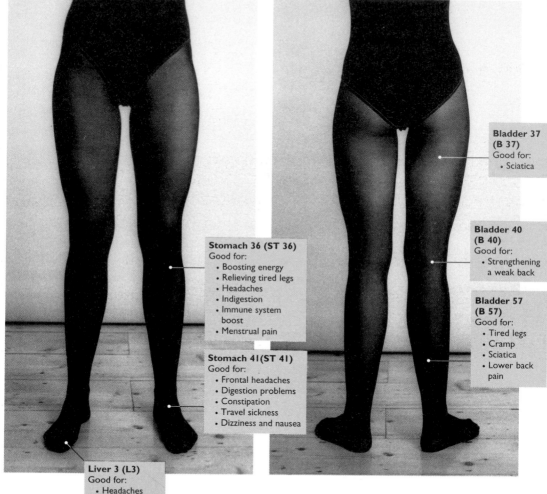

Bladder 37 (B 37)
Good for:
- Sciatica

Stomach 36 (ST 36)
Good for:
- Boosting energy
- Relieving tired legs
- Headaches
- Indigestion
- Immune system boost
- Menstrual pain

Bladder 40 (B 40)
Good for:
- Strengthening a weak back

Bladder 57 (B 57)
Good for:
- Tired legs
- Cramp
- Sciatica
- Lower back pain

Stomach 41(ST 41)
Good for:
- Frontal headaches
- Digestion problems
- Constipation
- Travel sickness
- Dizziness and nausea

Liver 3 (L3)
Good for:
- Headaches
- Menstrual pain
- Travel sickness
- Tight muscles
- Cramp

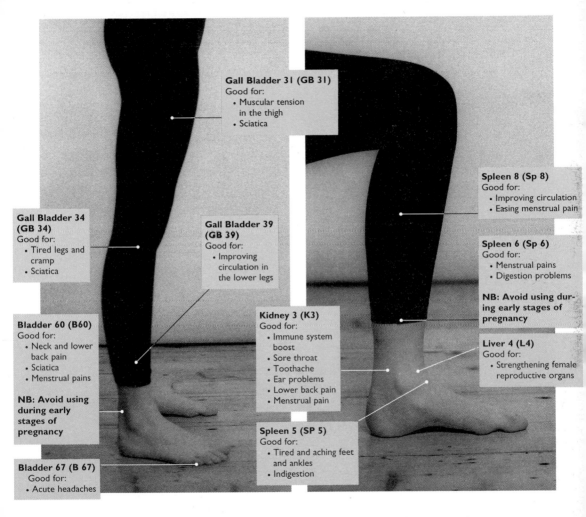

Gall Bladder 31 (GB 31)
Good for:
• Muscular tension in the thigh
• Sciatica

Spleen 8 (Sp 8)
Good for:
• Improving circulation
• Easing menstrual pain

Gall Bladder 34 (GB 34)
Good for:
• Tired legs and cramp
• Sciatica

Gall Bladder 39 (GB 39)
Good for:
• Improving circulation in the lower legs

Spleen 6 (Sp 6)
Good for:
• Menstrual pains
• Digestion problems

NB: Avoid using during early stages of pregnancy

Bladder 60 (B60)
Good for:
• Neck and lower back pain
• Sciatica
• Menstrual pains

NB: Avoid using during early stages of pregnancy

Kidney 3 (K3)
Good for:
• Immune system boost
• Sore throat
• Toothache
• Ear problems
• Lower back pain
• Menstrual pain

Liver 4 (L4)
Good for:
• Strengthening female reproductive organs

Bladder 67 (B 67)
Good for:
• Acute headaches

Spleen 5 (SP 5)
Good for:
• Tired and aching feet and ankles
• Indigestion

Doubling

FIVE MINUTE

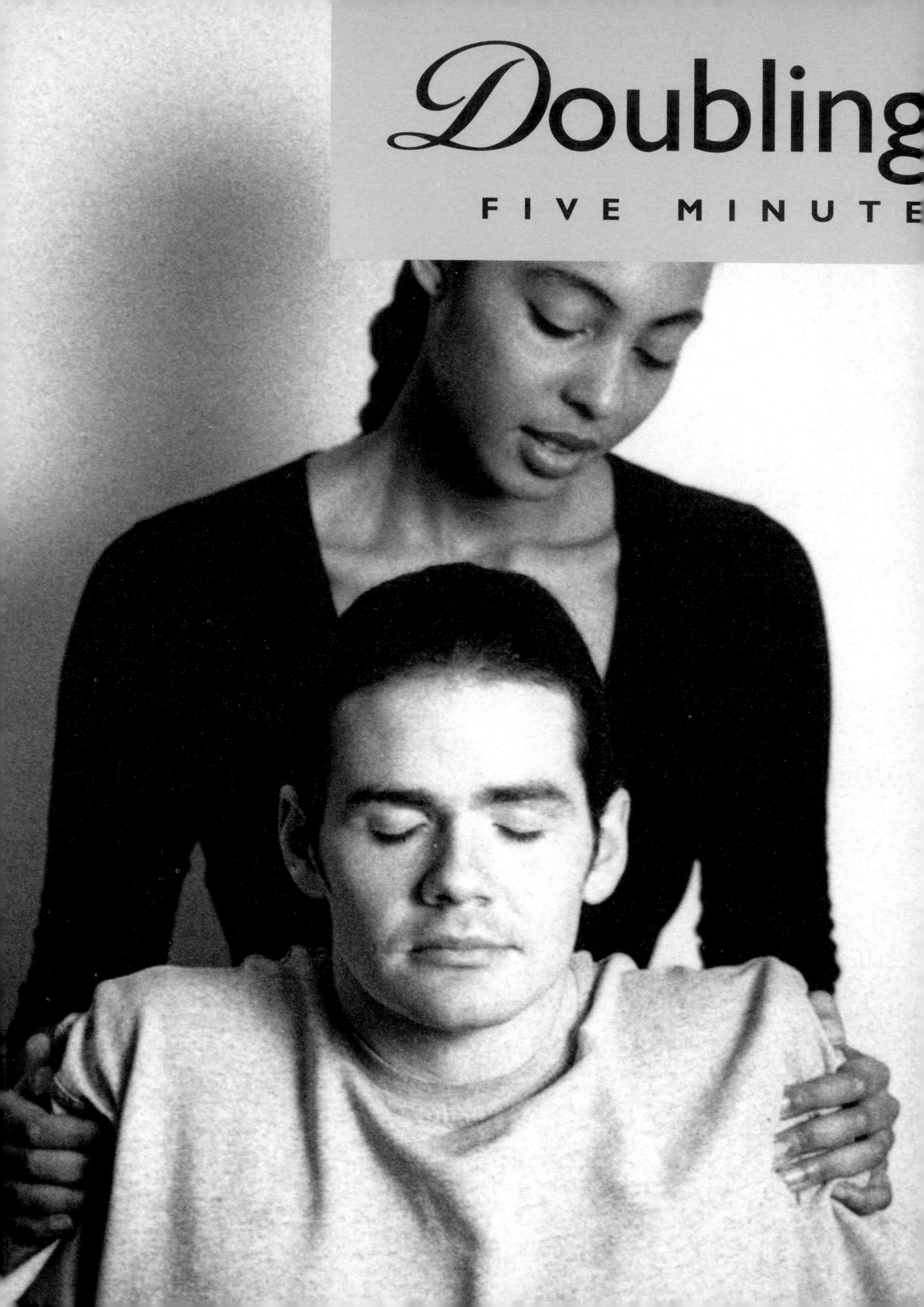

The Pleasure

MASSAGES FOR TWO

 *M*assaging yourself is an excellent way to learn about massage in general, since the feedback about where to work, what feels good, and how much pressure to use is immediate. However, sharing your skills with other people can bring a great deal of pleasure, not just for the person receiving but also for you, the giver.

Massage is one of the simplest gifts available. Through your fingers you can soothe away a difficult day, release tight, sore muscles, and allow the receiver to feel light and calm, recharged and more alive.

A few minutes and a positive caring attitude with a partner, a parent, a friend, a child or a work colleague can help bring an immediate change in the way that person feels, as well as creating trust and compassion between the two of you. This in itself is a small step towards improving your personal environment, and making the world a more peaceful and enjoyable place to live in.

Through the power of touch, you *can* make a difference.

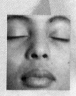

*W*orking with the head can be very calming and relaxing, particularly after a busy day. Make sure your partner is comfortable before you begin, and take a moment to calm yourself as well. Approach your partner slowly and keep your initial touch light and gentle. As they get used to your hands, you can begin to work with a firmer pressure.

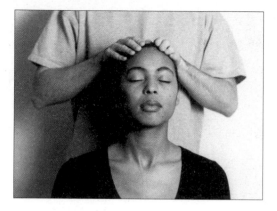

I Begin by positioning yourself behind your partner and gently stroke your hands through the hair with a smooth, unhurried rhythm to relax him or her.

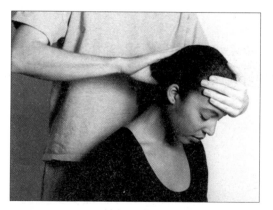

4 Place one hand on the forehead and ask your partner to let their head fall forward into your hand. Make sure you are supporting the full weight of the head, and place your thumb in the little hollow in the middle of the back of the skull. This is the Power Point Governing Vessel 16 (GV16). Make a small circle with the thumb and then press gently into the skull. Repeat several times along the bony ridge on left side up to the ear and then along the right.

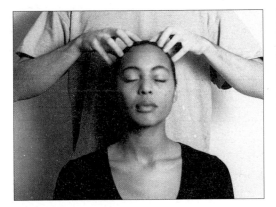

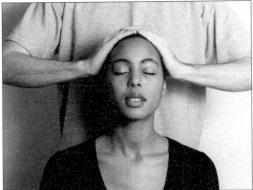

2 Then place the pads of your fingers on top of the scalp and move them in small circles. This area often gets very tight, but as you work you should feel the skin loosening up beneath your fingers. You can then swap and work even larger areas by using the palms of your hands.

3 Put your hands on either side of your partner's temples. Let the fingers rest on top of the head and gently press inwards with the heels. Release and move your hands further along the side and squeeze again, keeping the pressure light. Repeat until you reach just behind the ears. This move releases a lot of tension around the sides of the head and also feels great.

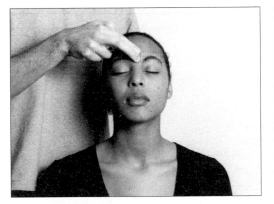

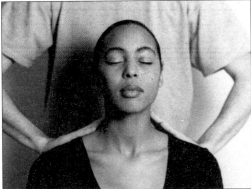

5 Bring the head back up and press the *Yintang* point which is located in the middle of the eyebrows; this releases a lot of tension in the face.

6 Finish by brushing down from the top of the head to the ends of the shoulders. Return to the top of the head and brush down to the bottom of the neck. Allow your partner a few moments to enjoy the effects of the session, and then check to see how they are.

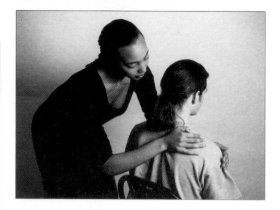

The neck and shoulders are a major trouble spot in the body, and most people love being massaged here.

I Begin by placing your left arm across your partner's chest for support, and then use the heel of your right hand to make large circles on the right shoulder. This feels good and is excellent for loosening up the shoulder muscles. After the right side is warmed up, change arms and work with the other side.

The secret to good massage is to learn to think with your fingers. This means clearing your mind, working mostly in silence, and letting your fingers explore your partner's muscles, searching for tightness. Not having to worry about what to do and whether you know the 'right thing', allows your fingers to work intuitively.

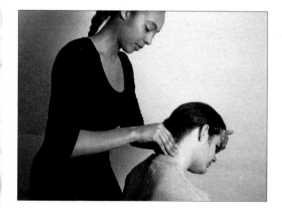

4 Still supporting the head, place your free hand on the neck and gently bring your fingers and thumb to the centre of the neck while still maintaining contact with the flesh. This can be very relaxing.

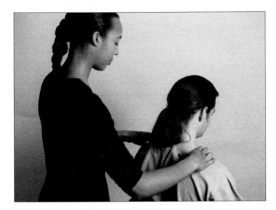

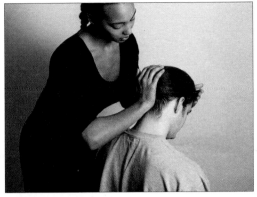

2 Then place both your thumbs at the top of the shoulders, and press into the muscles. Slowly begin to trace small circles with your thumbs, working across the shoulders in a T shape, first moving across, then back to the centre, and finally working downwards to loosen tight muscles between the shoulder blades.

3 Now that the shoulders have been loosened up, we can start to work on the neck, which is a key tension spot for practically everybody. Place one hand on the forehead, and ask your partner to drop the full weight of the head into your hand. Then place the heel of your hand on the back of the skull, push up gently, and begin to rub along the ridge. This should generate a feeling of warmth and also help to release a lot of the tension that accumulates in the muscles here.

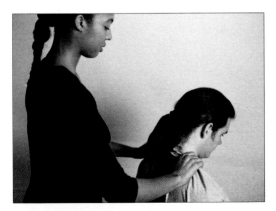

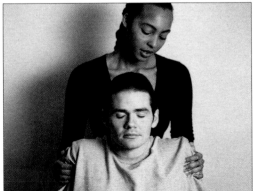

5 Returning to the shoulders, place both hands on either side of the neck and give them a big, firm squeeze. Make sure you don't pinch your partner, though! Work your way along the shoulders and repeat a few times.

6 Ask your partner to breathe in, and pick the shoulders up by the side arm muscles. Then ask him or her to breathe out and let go. Repeat this a few times and check with your partner, who should now be feeling a lot looser and more energized!

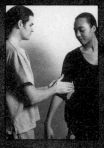

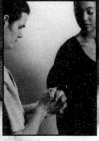

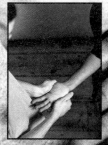

𝒯he arms and hands are a very safe place to work if you don't know a person too well, or they are apprehensive about being touched. Working here feels very relaxing and releases a lot of tension in the body. Be sure to ask your partner as you work whether they want firmer or lighter pressure. This will help to ensure the session is really enjoyable.

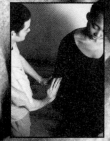

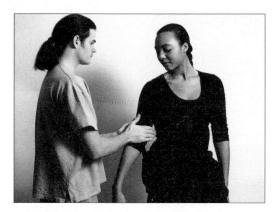

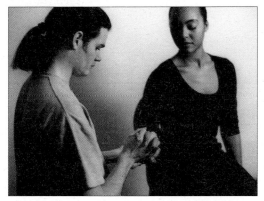

1 Take your partner's arm between your two hands and gently begin to roll and shake it. This really encourages the person to relax and let go of any tension. Work your way downwards and repeat.

2 Support your partner's arm with one hand and then interlace the fingers of their hand with yours. Firmly holding the hand, take the wrist through a gentle 360° rotation. This will increase the overall flexibility of the wrist. If you feel any spot where it seems to be 'sticky' or less flexible, continue to rotate the wrist until it loosens up. You can vary this by changing directions as well.

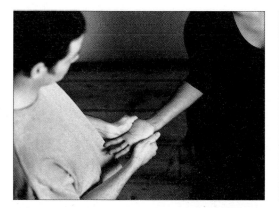

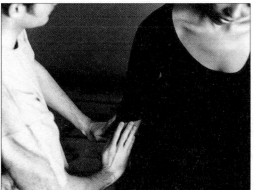

3 Place your fingers underneath your partner's hand and use your palms to open and stretch it. Adjectives used by people describing this experience include delicious and gorgeous, so don't hurry this.

4 Finally, place your hands at the top of the arm. Now lightly brush down to the fingertips and return to the top. Repeat several times, making sure you brush down all the sides of the arm. Your partner should now be feeling relaxed and may even report tingling feelings in the arms and hands. Repeat on the other arm.

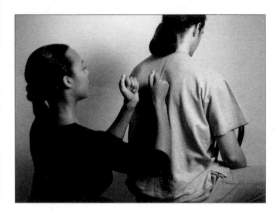

Form loose fists and gently pound your partner's back, starting at the top of the shoulders and then progressively working down the whole of the back. This helps to relax the back and prepare it for further work. Be careful not to pound directly on the spine, and to keep the pressure light especially towards the bottom of the back where the kidneys are located.

Everyone enjoys having a back massage since there are always areas of the back which need loosening up. One convenient way to work is to get your partner to straddle a chair and put some pillows between the back of the chair and his or her chest. Encourage your partner to relax and sink into the chair. While you work, make sure that you remain relaxed by keeping your shoulders down and breathing normally.

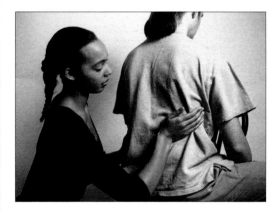

4 Return to making circles with your hand, but this time explore the rest of the back area. If you want you can also use your hand to work directly on the muscles which run alongside the spine (the erector spinae). Push them slightly away from the spine with the heel of the hand and then release. 'Twanging' the muscles like this feels good, and can also help loosen the whole back.

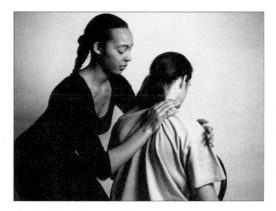

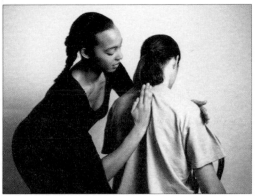

2 Next place your left arm across your partner's chest for support and using the heel of your hand, begin to make large circles in the shoulder area. Work one side thoroughly, then change arms and work the other side.

3 Supporting your partner still, use the edge of your hand to rub along the border of the shoulder blade, searching for tightness and congestion. This is a key area which is often very constricted, and responds quickly to being massaged. Then work the other side.

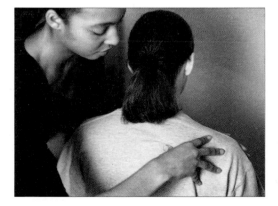

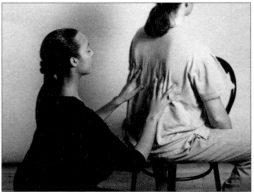

5 Support your partner again, and gently press your thumb into the muscle at the top of the shoulder about an inch away from the spine. Work in a straight line to the bottom of the back, and repeat on the other side.

6 Finally, form loose fists again and begin to pound the whole back once more. This will help to stimulate the back and also leave your partner feeling energized. Finish by brushing down the back a few times, and then check with your partner to see how they feel.

*A*fter a busy day, there is nothing better than having all the stresses and strains soothed away with a leg and foot massage. Follow these instructions while you work, but feel free to use your intuition and spend extra time on any areas that you feel could benefit from some extra attention and care.

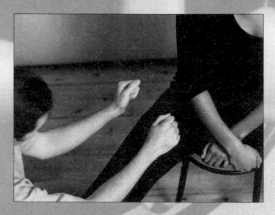

| Take one of your partner's legs and gently begin to pummel it with a loose fist. This will wake and energize the entire leg.

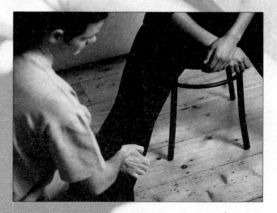

4 Support your partner's leg and gently massage the outside of the leg using the heel of your hand. Start at the top and work your way down. This can be tender so don't be too vigorous.

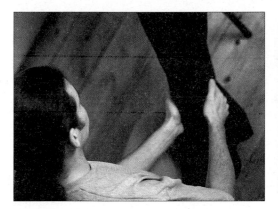

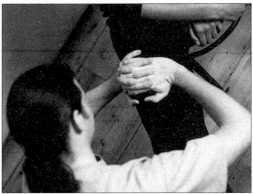

2 Then use both hands to cradle the top of the thigh. Begin a slow rocking movement from side to side, working your way right down to the lower leg. This helps the muscles to relax and feels very pleasant for the receiver.

3 Interlock your fingers. Then rest your hands on the thigh muscles near the top and squeeze the palms together. Release and move them slightly lower and repeat, working the whole thigh.

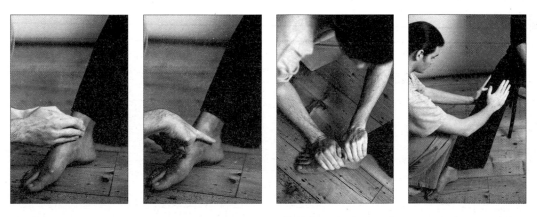

5 Then begin to work the ankle joint using your fingertips and massaging in small circles. Next use your index fingers to work just underneath the bones of the ankle, which feels very soothing.

6 Follow this by gently squeezing the top of the foot with the palm of your hand a few times. Brush down and repeat on the other leg.

A I L M E N T S   C H A R T

This chart is an invaluable companion in keeping you healthy and in optimum condition. It lists some of the major common ailments together with specific Power Points which can be of help in alleviating the symptoms. A variety of Power Points are given for each ailment so that you can choose only one or use all of them to maximize your body's own healing capability. Please note that the Power Points are not designed to replace orthodox medicine and that if your symptoms continue without any improvement you should consult your doctor for further advice and treatment.

ENERGY BOOSTERS

Head	pg 26	Governing Vessel 20
Wrist	pg 52	Triple Heater 4**
Hand	pg 53	Heart Governor 8
Leg	pg 80	Stomach 36

IMMUNE SYSTEM BOOSTERS

Hand	pg 52	Large Intestine 4**
Leg	pg 80	Stomach 36
Ankle	pg 81	Kidney 3

REDUCING STRESS AND TENSION

Head	pg 26	Governing Vessel 20
Back of Skull		
	pg 40	Governing Vessel 16
	pg 40	Gall Bladder 20
Arm	pg 53	Heart 3
Wrist	pg 53	Heart 7
Hand	pg 53	Heart Governor 8

REDUCING MUSCULAR TENSION

Leg	pg 81	Gall Bladder 34
Foot	pg 80	Liver 3

PAIN RELIEF

Back of Skull		
	pg 52	Large Intestine 4**
Arm	pg 52	Triple Heater 14

COLDS

Back of Skull		
	pg 40	Gall Bladder 20
Arm	pg 53	Lung 4
	pg 52	Triple Heater 5
	pg 53	Large Intestine 11
Wrist	pg 53	Lung 9
Hand	pg 53	Lung 10
	pg 53	Lung 11
	pg 52	Large Intestine 4**
	pg 53	Heart Governor 8

POOR CIRCULATION

Arm	pg 53	Large Intestine 10
Hand	pg 52	Triple Heater 4
Legs	pg 81	Gall Bladder 39

TRAVEL SICKNESS AND NAUSEA

Arm	pg 53	Heart Governor 6
Wrist	pg 53	Heart Governor 7
Leg	pg 80	Stomach 41
Foot	pg 80	Liver 3

HEADACHES/MIGRAINES

Face	pg 26	Yintang
	pg 26	Bladder 1
	pg 26	Bladder 2
	pg 27	Gall Bladder 12
Back of Skull		
	pg 40	Governing Vessel 16
	pg 40	Bladder 10
	pg 40	Gall Bladder 20
Wrist	pg 52	Large Intestine 5
	pg 52	Triple Heater 5
Leg	pg 80	Stomach 41
	pg 80	Stomach 36
Foot	pg 80	Liver 3
	pg 81	Bladder 67

EYESTRAIN

Head	pg 26	Yintang
	pg 26	Bladder1
	pg 26	Bladder 2
	pg 26	Stomach 1
Back of Skull		
	pg 40	Gall Bladder 20
Wrist	pg 52	Large Intestine 5
	pg 52	Triple Heater 5

EARACHE

Face	pg 27	Triple Heater 21
	pg 27	Small Intestine 19
Wrist	pg 52	Triple Heater 5
Feet	pg 81	Kidney 3

SINUS CONGESTION

Face	pg 26	Bitong
	pg 26	Large Intestine 20
	pg 26	Stomach 3
Back of Skull		
	pg 40	Governing Vessel 16
	pg 40	Gall Bladder 20
Arm	pg 53	Large Intestine 11
Wrist	pg 53	Lung 9
Hand	pg 52	Large Intestine 4**
	pg 53	Lung 10
	pg 53	Lung 11
	pg 52	Large Intestine 1

JAW ACHE

Face	pg 27	Gall Bladder 2

TOOTHACHE

Face	pg 27	Gall Bladder 2
Hand	pg 52	Large Intestine 4**
Wrist	pg 52	Large Intestine 5
Ankle	pg 81	Kidney 3

SORE THROAT

Back of Skull		
	pg 40	Gall Bladder 20
Wrist	pg 53	Lung 9
	pg 52	Large Intestine 5
Hand	pg 52	Large Intestine 4**
	pg 53	Lung 11
Foot	pg 81	Kidney 3

COUGHS

Chest	pg 66	Lung 1
Arm	pg 53	Lung 4
	pg 66	Lung 5

NECK TENSION/PAIN

Back of skull		
	pg 40	Gall Bladder 20
Back	pg 67	Bladder 12
	pg 67	Bladder 13
	pg 67	Small Intestine 11
	pg 67	Small Intestine 14
	pg 67	Small Intestine 15
Arm	pg 52	Large Intestine 14
Wrist	pg 52	Small Intestine 5
	pg 52	Small Intestine 6
Ankle	pg 81	Bladder 60**

SHOULDER TENSION/PAIN

Back of Skull		
	pg 40	Gall Bladder 20
Shoulders		
	pg 40	Gall Bladder 21**
	pg 41	Large Intestine 15
	pg 41	Large Intestine 16
Back	pg 67	Small Intestine 11
	pg 67	Small Intestine 14
	pg 67	Small Intestine 15
Arm	pg 52	Triple Heater 14
	pg 52	Large Intestine 14
Wrist	pg 52	Small Intestine 5
	pg 52	Small Intestine 6

ARM TENSION/PAIN

Arms	pg 52	Large Intestine 14
	pg 52	Triple Heater 14
	pg 53	Large Intestine 11
Wrist	pg 52	Triple Heater 4
	pg 52	Small Intestine 5

WRIST TENSION/PAIN

Wrist	pg 52	Triple Heater 4
	pg 52	Triple Heater 5
	pg 52	Small Intestine 5
	pg 52	Small Intestine 6

CHEST PAINS

Chest	pg 66	Central Vessel 17
	pg 66	Lung 1
Wrist	pg 53	Heart 7
	pg 53	Lung 9
Hand	pg 53	Heart Governor 8

BREATHING DIFFICULTIES/ASTHMA

Chest	pg 66	Lung 1
	pg 66	Central Vessel 17
Abdomen		
	pg 66	Central Vessel 6
Arm	pg 53	Lung 4
Wrist	pg 53	Lung 9
Hand	pg 53	Lung 10

INDIGESTION/ABDOMINAL PAINS

Face	pg 26	Stomach 1
Arm	pg 53	Large Intestine 11
	pg 52	Large Intestine 14
Wrist	pg 53	Heart Governor 6
	pg 52	Small Intestine 5
Hand	pg 52	Small Intestine 3
	pg 52	Large Intestine 4**
Abdomen		
	pg 66	Stomach 25
Leg	pg 80	Stomach 36
	pg 81	Spleen 6**
	pg 80	Stomach 41
	pg 81	Spleen 5

CONSTIPATION

Arm	pg 53	Large Intestine 11
Abdomen		
	pg 66	Stomach 25
Leg	pg 80	Stomach 36
	pg 80	Stomach 41

MENSTRUAL PAINS

Abdomen		
	pg 66	Central Vessel 6
	pg 66	Central Vessel 4
Sacrum		
	pg 67	Bladder 26
	pg 67	Bladder 27
	pg 67	Bladder 28
	pg 67	Bladder 29
Hand	pg 52	Large Intestine 4**
	pg 53	Heart Governor 6
Leg	pg 80	Stomach 36
	pg 81	Spleen 8
	pg 81	Spleen 6**
Ankle	pg 81	Liver 4
	pg 81	Bladder 60**
	pg 81	Kidney 3
Foot	pg 80	Liver 3

LOWER BACK PAIN

Back	pg 67	Small Intestine 14
	pg 67	Small Intestine 15
Wrist	pg 52	Small Intestine 6
Knee	pg 80	Bladder 40
Leg	pg 80	Bladder 57
Ankle	pg 81	Kidney 3
	pg 81	Bladder 60**

SCIATICA

Sacrum		
	pg 67	Bladder 26
Buttocks		
	pg 67	Gall Bladder 30
Legs	pg 81	Gall Bladder 31
	pg 81	Gall Bladder 34
	pg 80	Bladder 37
	pg 80	Bladder 57
	pg 81	Bladder 60**

TIRED LEGS

Leg	pg 81	Gall Bladder 31
	pg 81	Gall Bladder 34
	pg 80	Bladder 57
	pg 80	Stomach 36

CRAMP

Leg	pg 81	Gall Bladder 34
	pg 80	Bladder 57

ANKLE TENSION/PAIN

Foot	pg 81	Spleen 5

TIRED/ACHING FEET

Foot	pg 81	Spleen 5

*** Do not use these points if you are trying to conceive or are pregnant - select a different point from the chart.*

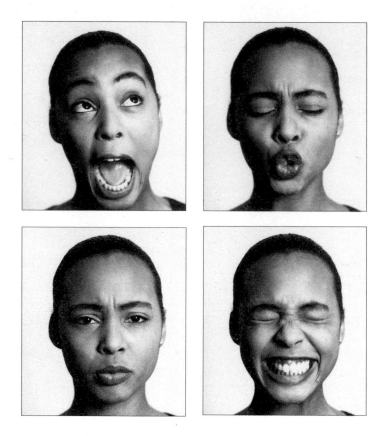